In Less Than One Month, You Can Transform Your Life!

Janet Greeson, Ph.D., is a nationally renowned pioneer in the development of addiction treatment programs. In this revised edition of her groundbreaking classic, she presents a refined and restructured 28-day plan to help you overcome hidden food addictions. Through nutrition, exercise, relaxation, and stress management, you'll learn how to reshape your attitudes as well as your body—how to live "happy, joyous, and free." Discover:

- The *10 Points of Positive Mental Attitude*
- Exercises to increase self-awareness and find the "Real Me" in you
- A fabulous new international cuisine, featuring delicious low-fat recipes
- Movement therapies to develop a positive body image
- Meditation, visualization, and other relaxation techniques
- The empowering support of a "buddy" system—and how to create one
- Case histories of food addicts who are in recovery from compulsive overeating, bulimia, and anorexia—to offer hope and help along the way

For anyone who ever feared that too much would never be enough, Janet Greeson's *IT'S NOT WHAT YOU'RE EATING, IT'S WHAT'S EATING YOU* is motivation, inspiration—and liberation—at last!

Books by Janet Greeson, Ph.D.

It's Not What You're Eating, It's What's Eating You
Food for Love

Published by POCKET BOOKS

IT'S NOT WHAT YOU'RE EATING, IT'S WHAT'S EATING YOU

JANET GREESON, Ph.D.

POCKET BOOKS

New York   London   Toronto   Sydney   Tokyo   Singapore

When God Becomes a Drug: Breaking the Chains of Religious Addiction and Abuse, Father Leo Booth, Putnam/Tarcher, © 1991. Reprinted with permission from Father Leo Booth.

Sex and Love Addiction: 40 Questions for Self-Diagnosis, © 1985. Reprinted with permission from the Augustine Fellowship, Sex and Love Addicts Anonymous.

POCKET BOOKS, a division of Simon & Schuster Inc.
1230 Avenue of the Americas, New York, NY 10020

ISBN: 0-671-86703-2

First Pocket Books paperback printing February 1994

10 9 8 7 6 5 4 3 2 1

POCKET and colophon are registered trademarks of
Simon & Schuster Inc.

Printed in the U.S.A.

Acknowledgments

"We can do no great things,
only little things with great love."

—*Mother Teresa*

No one can write a book alone. This book was made possible by the love of God and St. Teresa, "the little flower." It grew out of the combined support of precious friends who refused to give up on me, year after year. Their devotion and relentless energy go far beyond mere gratitude, but I will try.

First, Catherine Revland is holding a reservation for a front row seat in heaven, I'm sure of it. She's an angel. Without Catherine's wisdom, the following pages would still be dancing inside my head. She and God made it all make sense.

I am blessed to have the gentle, warm love, and intelligence of my mother reflected in these pages, and in my life. The strength, love, and bursting good humor of my children, Gene, Jimmy, and Roe, kept me going when I couldn't find anything funny. They have always been there for me and have made my life wonderfully exciting.

How very fortunate I am to have Budd Holden and Andre Piot as real friends who inspire me to remain "God's kid" always. I see God's love reflected in them every day with love, life, and truth.

Love is experienced in many ways, and because "Your Life Matters" is really God's company, He put wonderful angels in my life and on my staff. Kitty Duffy's love and trust, Marty Van Herik's warm friendship, Deneice Howard's compassion, Fred Earle's loving spirit, Beatrice Cohen's humor, Jann Seller's warmth, Bob Crane's spontaneity, Paige Hargrove's shining light, Kim Comeau's abundant energy, Jack Ayala's loving spark, Larry Dean's loyalty, Jerry Smith's dedication, Peggy Favata's kindness, Roland Mora's kindred spirit, and Tom Bell's love. Let me not forget past husbands who have made my life interesting and fun.

I will be forever grateful to my editor, Denise Silvestro, who captured this book in her own delicate and sensitive way, and appreciation always to my agent, Frank Weiman.

Special love to all present and past staff of "Your Life Matters" who have dedicated themselves to making a difference in the lives of others. You are all God's kids and you make the difference. I also thank Mother Teresa, Dr. Robert Schuller, Oprah, and Joan Rivers who have impacted my life indirectly, but in a remarkable way.

I dedicate this book to you. It's your book now! My dream is that it will empower you to be all that you can be.

Contents

III

Recovery One Day at a Time

Preface

Since the publication of the first edition of this book in 1990, I have received thousands of letters from readers telling me that I have saved their lives. I don't believe I have saved anybody's life, but I do believe the process of recovery is so exciting that it is possible to stimulate and nurture people into wanting to heal, grow, and enhance who they are.

There are many reasons for this new edition. One is to provide more stimulation and nurturing. For those of you who have already read the first edition, this is another leg on a wonderful journey of excitement, change, and the full expression of who you really are. For those of you who have not read the first edition, this book will be a brand-new experience, for it will redirect your focus from losing weight to gaining a meaningful life.

Another reason for this new edition involves the changes that have taken place in treatment programs to make them more effective. Twelve years ago, when I opened my first treatment center, my patient population was 80–90 percent men admitted for alcoholism. My patients today are 80–90 percent women admitted for depression. Over the past six years, as we tracked thousands of patients through treatment, we realized that the latter progressed through treatment in a way that was remarkably different from the former. The alcoholic's falsely exaggerated sense of self had to be broken through before any real work could be done. Depressed people, on the other hand, came into treatment with their self-esteem already shattered. Their identity needed to be built up, not broken down.

The goal of treatment is to bring patients to a peak experience in which unresolved issues from the past emerge so that the feelings around those issues can be experienced and expressed. While alcoholics tend to have one peak experience late in treatment, depressed patients tend to have two, one after the first week of treatment and a second, higher peak experience during the last week. In between is a valley of conflicts, nightmares, and sometimes painful self-revelations. But the reward is great, for that second peak experience is often a real breakthrough that frees up the patient's undeveloped core being. The twenty-eight-day program in this edition has been revised to reflect the new knowledge we have gained about treating the depressed patient and bringing about that valuable second peak experience.

The changes in the twenty-eight-day program in this new edition also reflect a heightened awareness of the benefits of therapeutic exercises. Six years of experience at "Your Life Matters" has increased the effectiveness of the activities we assign to guide patients through a peak experience. More than ever, I believe that taking positive action is invaluable, whether it is with a group or a buddy, or in solitude. The most effective of the new activities developed in our treatment centers have been added to this revised edition.

Yet another reason for this new edition is the profound change in the perception of the prevalence of child abuse in our society, particularly sexual abuse. When I disclosed my grandfather's incest five years ago, I anguished over whether I was doing the right thing, for at the time my disclosure verged on the unthinkable. Since then many people have come forward to talk about their experiences of abuse, and the social climate has changed incredibly fast: the unthinkable now verges on the commonplace. As a result, people are more willing today to confront their experiences and are more likely to be believed by their therapists.

And a final reason: a slow but widespread acceptance of the realization that diets don't work because they don't address the problem. This change in perception has been a long time coming, but at last attention is being paid to it. I am grateful, for this new perception allows us to focus on freeing ourselves from the prison we are in. Those of us who suffer from food addiction live in the prison of our own bodies. If you dislike or struggle with your body, you are in one, too. The prison is entrapping you in the false image you have of your body, an image no one else in the world sees but you. The tragedy of being in this prison is that the incarceration is not mandatory. You are in a state of self-imposed solitary confinement. You arrested yourself, you were the prosecuting attorney, the judge and the jury, and you are now the prison guard.

You built your prison with the tools of your own imagination, not to incarcerate but to protect yourself. Your building blocks were painful memories and negative messages you picked up from other people and from society at large. You compared yourself to others, and to the impossible standards given to you by the media, and found yourself lacking. Although everyone has flaws, you saw yours alone.

You fortify those walls every day with new messages of negativity, not just from others but from yourself, and your own criticism is the harshest of all. You reject messages of acceptance and love because they do not fit into the structure you have built for yourself.

Is it any wonder that people who suffer from food addiction are deeply depressed? In fact, unhappiness is the universal symptom expressed by people who come to my treatment centers. But through my experiences I have come to realize that depression is not a symptom of food addiction, but rather at the root of the problem. I used to weigh 350 pounds, and I always felt that my body was all anyone could see. This negative image was reinforced by people around me; whenever I went to the doctor, whether I had the flu, asthma, or a broken leg, it seemed as though the physician would always wind up discussing my weight. It was only years later that I discovered that a combination of fear, anger, and depression was my real problem. I was using food to kill myself in a slow, numb way.

The stories within these pages are not about food but about broken hearts, broken dreams, how life becomes a struggle, and about people who, no matter what they try to do, feel stuck in their mental prison. You can't treat food addiction by focusing on the food; that's like applying a Band-Aid to a deep, festering wound. And every new diet is just a different bandage; it might work for a while, or at least mask the wound, but the most beautiful Band-Aid in the world is not going to heal it.

The body heals itself from the inside out, never the other way around. The only way to treat a deep wound is to go to the root of it, as painful as that may be, clean it out, and apply a nurturing dressing. Given the right attention, the body miraculously heals itself, and when the bandages are removed, there may be no sign at all of the damage that was there. No scars.

The wounded mind heals in a similar way. Broken dreams can be mended, once the damage that has been done is cleaned out at its deepest source. Even the wounds of childhood can be healed. My mission is to make a difference in your life by helping you mend your dreams, from the inside out, so you can walk about freely, bouncing with life.

Deeply wounded people are desperate; they are willing to try almost anything to relieve their pain. They go on every new diet that comes along, or try intense exercise programs, but still no healing takes place. Diet and exercise are important, but they treat only the symptoms. Even therapy alone does not work; when the mind alone is treated, people can stay imprisoned in their thoughts forever, intellectualizing but never experiencing what they feel. In treating thousands of patients I have come to believe that no single approach will work. The mind and body must work together. The mind is capable of telling us incredible lies, convincing us that merely thinking about something is experiencing it. For instance, people can talk about their anger and never really feel it; but when mind and body work together, a catharsis takes place. By simultaneously expressing anger (feeling) with action (body movement) as well as words (mind), you can truly experience anger, often for the first time, as well as experience the relief that comes when a strong and sometimes terrifying emotion is discharged. This book is designed to get the mind and body working together; the exercises for each day will help you to experience life.

Many readers have told me they use this book not just with a buddy, as I recommend, but in discussion with friends they have come to trust in ways that enhance their relationships. Although it is possible to derive much benefit from working with a buddy alone, I enthusiastically support taking advantage of a group effort, if it is available. After many years of treating people with depression, I now have statistical data confirming my belief that no single approach to treatment will ever be as powerful as a group effort. It's amazing how the combined energy of a group can bring everyone in the group to a higher level of mind. But remember this: Whether you choose to work with a buddy or a group, recovery takes action, and without it people are likely to remain prisoners of their own thoughts forever.

I have come into your life to help you plot your escape from the prison you may be in. You don't need a saw or a crowbar, for you are in possession of the key that will unlock the prison door. Healing begins with love, not from without, but from within. Love of self will unlock the prison door. It may not open easily after being shut for so long, but your imagination, which put you where you are, can also set you free.

The sun is shining outside the prison walls, and the breezes are gently blowing. What are you waiting for? Let's go!

I

It's Not What You're Eating

1

I Am Not My Body

Please allow me to make an assumption about you. You are reading this book because you are unhappy about your relationship with food. What was once a source of enjoyment now gives you pain. Intrigued by the title, you have begun reading to look for the answer you have never found in the many diet books you have read: mainly, why you can't eat like "normal" people. You have picked up this book because sooner or later (mostly sooner) your willpower fails and food controls your thoughts and your actions, and even haunts your dreams. You have picked it up because you suspect that, yes, there something definitely is "eating me."

Before we begin, it's very important that you leave behind all the concepts about food and dieting you've read elsewhere. My approach is so different that before I begin to explain it, I feel the need to reorient you in a totally new direction.

IT'S NOT WHAT YOU'RE EATING

This is not a book about food; it's about feelings. It's not about the stuffing, it's about the stuffee. It's not about how much you eat or what you eat or don't eat, or how often you eat, but what happens to you when you do eat. Any weight loss plan that does not uncouple feelings from food is bound to fail. This is a book for people who eat not to nourish their bodies but to make themselves *feel* better. It is the first book to treat the use of food as a mood-altering substance, as an addiction.

Food addiction is a disease of the human spirit, and it can't be cured by a physical solution alone. Trying to do so is nearly as painful as leaving it untreated.

Don't be frightened by the idea that you might have a disease. Broken down, the word reveals its simple meaning: dis-ease, or the absence of comfort. Acknowledging you have a disease permits dignity and the right to obtain medical attention for something that is *not your fault*. It banishes all ideas of guilt, lack of control, and even the word "diet," which beyond the first explanatory chapter you will not even find in this book.

THREE REASONS WHY DIETS DON'T WORK

It's true you can lose weight on them, sometimes a lot. The problem is gaining all those pounds back again, plus a few extra, which is all but inevitable. I know someone who lost a hundred pounds in six months on the Dr. Atkins diet and gained them all back in six weeks! Very few dieters manage to sustain a weight loss, particularly a dramatic one.

You undoubtedly know diets don't work, but think the reason is your lack of willpower. That's like blaming diabetics for their inability to metabolize sugar. The reason diets don't work has nothing to do with self-restraint and everything to do with body chemistry and the way the mind functions.

First, the physical aspect: The body can handle only one extended fast in a lifetime. Sudden or prolonged deprivation of food lowers its metabolism rate, which is the amount of calories it requires to burn each day in order to function. In the millions of years human beings have existed, this metabolic adjustment served an important evolutionary purpose. During periods of famine, it assured the survival of those whose bodies were ingesting fewer calories.

Because of our heritage, crash diets are self-defeating. They trigger our genetic alarm system, decreasing the amount of calories we need to function and causing our bodies to store extra fat as a hedge against future deprivation, thus keeping us a prisoner of calorie-counting forever. Fortunately, all is not lost. Exercise and proper nutrition will eventually restore our metabolism rate somewhat, though it's debatable if we will ever get back to where we started. Obviously, the sensible thing is never to go on a crash fasting diet in the first place.

The second reason diets fail occurs in the mind. Have you ever noticed that as soon as you go on a diet, you start obsessing about food more than ever? The reason is simple: People move toward their most dominant thought, even if that thought is about not having something. Diets are all about deprivation. Even the word sets up a bad connotation: "die-et," or as a psychologist friend of mine defines it, "You die because you et." Go on a diet and you'll start dying for whatever it is you crave, because you can't have it. Suddenly, all your mental energy is expended on fulfillment of that one dominant thought. As a result, even while managing to resist putting the forbidden food into your mouth, you're still a prisoner of food in your mind. You might not be burning the calories, but your mind is burning with thoughts about what you're not eating. No wonder diets make people so depressed!

In this book, I will not talk about diets. I will talk about food plans. Instead of focusing on deprivation, we will focus on what you *can* eat, and I'm sure you will find there are a lot of foods you like in the daily menus listed here.

The third reason diets don't work is that they focus on control. Because people with eating disorders think in terms of controlling what they eat, they are often very rigid in their attitude. After all, addiction to food is much more difficult to live with than addiction to alcohol or other substances from which people can totally abstain. There's an Overeaters Anonymous (or OA) saying: "You can put the plug in the jug and keep it there, but you've got to take the tiger out of the cage three times a day and feed it without getting hurt." Because eating is necessary to life, food addicts often believe they must control the urge to eat to excess every time they put food in their mouths, but sooner or later that negativity will do them in and they'll attack food with a vengeance.

We've all had what we consider *bad* foods. Notice how we put moral labels on food. We give it such power. I tell myself, just because I made a mistake doesn't mean I *am* a mistake. In dealing with food, we're all going to make mistakes. The problem with most dieting is that people think because the diet is a failure, they're a failure. As hard as they try, and as motivated as they are, they just don't know how to exercise control over food.

There is a widespread myth about food addicts that control is their main issue. I disagree. Control is a symptom. The core issue is powerlessness. The food addict gives away the power to the food. Think of the power people give to that "just one" potato chip that will lead to a binge.

I don't believe in focusing on control. It makes as much sense as treating an allergic rash with a skin cream. You don't treat the symptom, you treat the addiction, and the addiction is about powerlessness. Instead of encouraging you to increase your willpower, I will encourage you to embrace your powerlessness. In order to conquer food addiction you do not conquer it:

"What you resist persists."* Going into battle with food gives it power, because it becomes a moral issue. That's why it's a mistake to label food good or bad; if people eat "bad" food, they tend to think they become bad themselves. As a consequence they may do penance, and sometimes the punishment they mete out is eating more, or doing without, which puts them back into the deprivation mode again.

We live in a society of learned helplessness. All our lives people tell us we can't do things, and we grow up giving away our power by learning to rely on someone else or society to have all the answers. My goal in this book is to encourage you to claim your own power. This may seem impossible at this point, but believe me, it will work for you as it has for me and many thousands of others.

Fifteen years ago I weighed 340 pounds and had been dieting half my life, losing the same 100 pounds over and over again. I was not so much living as existing, and knew I was eating myself to death. I lost the weight I needed to lose and kept it off—permanently—not by dieting. I have a food plan called 301—three meals a day, nothing in between, and one day at a time—and I follow a program that requires me to make major changes not so much in my eating habits as in my attitudes and my behavior. Although I will remain a food addict until the day I die, I am no longer a prisoner of my body, and that has liberated my mind from obsession and allowed me to create a full, rich, and happy life for myself. You can, too.

---

*Unattributed quotes that appear in boldface in this book are 12-step axioms, which, like the program, are anonymous.

FOOD AS AN ADDICTION

You are probably still uncomfortable with the term "food addict." When I use the word "addiction," I mean the continued use of a mood-altering substance in spite of the negative consequences, coupled with a greatly diminished capacity to exercise free will over its use. Addiction is characterized by overdoing, in spite of lost health, jobs, relationships, and status. If there are no negative consequences to your behavior in relation to food, and if there is no disparity between your need to control your intake of food and your ability to do so, then you aren't an addict. If there is, I hope you will keep an open mind and consider the fact that you might be one.

Another helpful definition of addiction comes from the "Big Book" of Alcoholics Anonymous: "a mental obsession coupled with a physical compulsion." Food addicts are constantly thinking about food and cannot stop eating once they start. That's the double whammy of the addiction; not only do your thoughts propel you to eat, physical changes take place when you eat that cause you to keep eating without the ability to stop when you're no longer hungry. An alcoholic can never understand how a person can sit and nurse one drink all night. A food addict can never understand how a person can cut a sliver out of a cake and not wind up eating the whole thing. And when that cake is gone, the food addict experiences no satisfaction, only disgust and shame. I relate that feeling to a cat's making love to a skunk: I didn't have all I wanted, but I had about all I could stand.

Because it is the earliest addiction, food is very often the primary one. Many alcoholics manage to stop drinking only to be confronted with their addiction to food in their recovery. It is also the most common addiction. More people die from it each year than from all the other addictions combined, yet there's rarely an emphasis put on food as a potentially lethal substance. There are no labels on bakery trucks or photos of seven-layer cakes in magazines that announce, "Warning: Consumption may be dangerous to your health." Nor is there much social stigma attached to food addiction. Eating too much is generally considered a joke, but I didn't laugh at the sign I recently saw on the wall of a New York restaurant: "*Morte de Pasta*—proudly killing you since 1985."

GENETIC ADDICTION

Food addiction runs in families. Women tend to abuse food more than men, who tend to turn to alcohol instead. Mothers who abuse food pass on their addiction to their children. If one or both of your parents were food addicts, the chances are great that you're one, too. A significant amount of medical research has been conducted on the theory that certain people are born addicted, so that by rights a biopsy could be done at birth to determine whether a person was going to grow up to be an addict. Not every addict is genetically addicted, but those of us who are have fewer of the chemical brain messengers known as endorphins, and that deficiency causes us to feel as if we're always "running on low." Certain mood-altering substances such as sugar, alcohol, opiates, and other drugs penetrate the blood barrier of the brain, causing a feeling of euphoria, which is intensified in the genetically addicted, for they are accustomed to feeling "low."

The molecular structures of sugar and alcohol are similar when they are broken down in the body. Because of their special neurochemical sensitivity, addicts develop an allergy to sugar that triggers a vicious cycle of craving: at first, eating sweets does make them feel better by raising their blood sugar, but when it drops again, the body cries out for more, repeating the cycle. Stress also triggers a sugar craving, causing mind-altering chemicals such as catecholamine to stimulate the appetite. People eat a sweet snack to relieve the stress, and after the sugar drop-off, they're back in the cycle of craving again. Heavy carbohydrate meals can also lead to sugar consumption. They trigger release of the chemical brain-messenger serotonin, an endorphin that reduces mental alertness. Then, when people get drowsy, they turn to sugar again for a quick pick-me-up. Because of its prevalence in society, and its connection to the joys of childhood, sugar is rarely seen as the drug it really is.

Some people are born endorphin deficient. From the very first time they ingest substances that raise their abnormally low endorphin levels, they feel a tremendous sense of well-being. With the continued use of a substance the addiction cycle has begun. Food addicts can vividly recall the special foods of their childhood, alcoholics that first drink; and you'd be amazed at the intensity of the memory.

INCREASED TOLERANCE

Unfortunately, you never have enough of what you want, because the substance is not what you really want—it's the feeling. In addition, that initial euphoria cannot be sustained, for addiction is a progressive disease. As time goes on, it takes more and more food to sustain an increasingly diminishing intensity level of feeling good. Eventually that wonderful feeling of well-being that makes the early stages of addiction so seductive becomes a source of disenchantment, for it is never reached again, no matter how much of the mood-altering substance is taken. The first time an alcoholic drinks, he might get a buzz after two drinks. Later it will take six or seven to get comparatively high. In advanced stages he might drink the whole bottle and feel nothing at all.

The same increased tolerance takes place in food addicts. In the early stages, a few slices of cake will produce the good feelings they seek, then half the cake, and pretty soon, the whole thing. In advanced stages not even that gives them the intensity of feeling they crave. No matter what or how much they eat, they get no relief. Everyone has abused food at some time in his or her life, but when people have to eat more and more to elevate their mood or, as the disease progresses, to achieve a soporific numbness, you're looking at addiction. With today's increased awareness and education about fitness and nutrition, if overeating were just a bad habit, we would be making terrific strides, but we're not. The United States has the largest population of overeaters in the world. Even our children's percentage of body fat has increased.

The same pattern of increased tolerance is true for anorexics. They eat less and less, looking for the intensity. Bulimics often complain that they feel numb, saying the only time they feel intensely is when they vomit. It gets them high, but after a while even that violent experience leaves them feeling numb.

WITHDRAWAL

Another sign of addiction is the state of discomfort a person experiences in the absence of the substance of choice. Nicotine addicts who light up a cigarette first thing in the morning are in a state of withdrawal, having not ingested their drug since the night before, and they need it just to start their day. Sugar withdrawal, which people experience when they go on a diet, produces headaches, listlessness, and irritability as intense as other kinds of drug detoxification. It's one of the reasons why going on a diet is such a miserable experience. People who are ravenously hungry right before bed, three or four hours after a big dinner, or who get up in the middle of the night to raid the refrigerator, are also going through withdrawal. The intensity of their need has nothing to do with actual hunger. If true hunger were being experienced, that intensity would be appropriate after a night's sleep, or a busy morning of work. Looking for the times during the day when you are experiencing the greatest desire for food is a good way to determine whether that desire is out of real need or whether you're experiencing withdrawal.

ISOLATION

In the words of Robert Morley, "No man is lonely while eating spaghetti." That perfectly describes the relationship addicts have with their substance of choice. Addicts are emotional loners. Their feelings are attached to food, booze, drugs, work, other people, gambling, or whatever their obsessive–compulsive behavior uses as a distraction from their inner emptiness. Their energy is inner directed only with regard to the substance and outer directed only to the extent that they need others to tell them how they should look, feel, or think. Inside, there is a void where their own spirit should be. All their relationships are distorted. The food, the alcohol, the drugs, are always in between them and the relationship.

Addiction is a disease of isolation. Instead of having relationships with other people, the food addict withdraws from social contact to have a relationship with food. It isn't necessary to be alone to experience isolation. In fact, loneliness can be the most intense when one is surrounded by other people, none of whom the addict can feel close to. Intimacy is not possible when the people who desire closeness are not in touch with who they really are. In fact, they feel uncomfortable when they try to get close to others, and even when others think they are achieving intimacy, the addict knows it's not the real thing. Out of touch with their own authenticity, they feel like impostors. Frustrated in their attempts to seek intimacy with people, they try to have a love affair with food. The food calls to them. It has warmth. It is capable of nurturing. It lives! The problem of having a love affair with food is that it never satisfies. No amount will ever fill the emptiness inside.

IT'S WHAT'S EATING YOU

Food addicts are eating a whole lot more than food. They're eating feelings associated with food. If they're angry, they'll go for a crunchy food. If they're in need of mothering, they'll go for something soft, sweet, and milky. There's a well-known laboratory experiment that illustrates this linkage of food and feelings. A mother monkey died, and her babies were dying because they would not take milk from a bottle. The scientists made a wire-mesh monkey and covered it with fur, then fed the baby monkeys through the wire mesh so they could get warmth and nurturing along with their food. All the babies flourished. Food addicts are like those baby monkeys. The connection between food and comfort is so deep they can't make the distinction. They go for food instead of going after what they really want, which is intimacy with people.

Food addicts will often develop cravings around food associated with early nurturing. For me it was mashed potatoes. My father loved them, and we had them every day. As a grown woman, when I craved them, they weren't just mashed potatoes; they stood for love, nurturing, and security. Addicts have trouble sorting out the source of these feelings, particularly pleasurable ones that they find hard to accept and have to distort. Deep down, they really don't believe they deserve to feel good. When they do, they worry that they're not going to get enough of those good feelings, or they come into contact with how needy they are, and that neediness scares them. Because their lives are so full of stress and crises, when they do feel pleasure, they don't know how to relax and enjoy it without feeling guilty.

Food addicts will readily tell you what they think, but they have a hard time telling you what they feel. After so many years of denying their emotions, the only way they can feel is through the eating, denial, or purging of food. A binge is really an explosion of emotion. As soon as bingers grasp that concept, they can use identification of feelings as an intervention when the power of the urge to binge overcomes them. They can allow themselves to experience their feelings so they can express them rather than feed them more food.

Sooner or later food loses its ability to dull the pain of unexpressed feelings. Turning to it or any other substance for solace is seeking your identity from the outside, where it can never be found. The form your addiction takes really doesn't matter. It's the content, namely your emptiness, that matters, that void you feel you have to fill up with someone or something outside of yourself to feel complete.

HITTING BOTTOM

Hitting bottom is that moment when food no longer alters your state of mind, and you really feel the depths of your anguish. Reality glares like a spotlight on the truth of your situation, illuminating what you've been trying so hard to deny—that your life is unmanageable, that you're both helpless and hopeless, and can find no way out of your pain short of dying.

No one else can measure that pain. It can't be calibrated by whether you have two hundred pounds to lose or twenty. If those extra pounds are making you miserable, damaging your self-esteem and your ability to cope with life, or if you're keeping your normal weight by secret vomiting, or if you're so thin, people are alarmed while your mind is still telling you you're fat, the pain is all the same—unmeasurable. Only you know when you've taken all the pain you can stand.

Be glad you've hit bottom, because once you've arrived at that despairing place, you can change. Your chances for recovery are actually greater than those for people who don't feel desperate. There's a Zen saying, "When the student is ready, the teacher appears." Once you've acknowledged you don't have the answer, you open yourself up to the possibility of seeking an answer elsewhere—one that *does* work. Hitting bottom isn't the end of the world. It's the anteroom to a new one. It's not a tragedy. It's an epiphany.

GETTING HELP

It may be no accident this book appeared in your life at this particular time. If you're ready to get help, you can determine what kind of help you need at the end of this chapter, where there is a quiz you can take. It will help you determine whether you're addicted to food. Going into treatment is the ultimate preparation for recovery, but that may not be possible for you in your present circumstances. I have written this book to serve as an alternative to treatment. If you commit yourself to following the steps laid out before you here, it will be the next best thing to experiencing a treatment center.

Merely reading this book, however, will not get you on the road to recovery. "You can't think yourself into good acting, but you can act yourself into good thinking." My program requires you to take action, even before you believe it will work for you. In fact, the addict in you will really rebel at first, and do everything to convince you that your new attempt is just another failure on your part. But if you ignore the voice of that powerful disease within you that is causing you so much pain, and take the simple actions required by this program, I'm telling you now you *will* succeed. I did, and you can, too.

Eighteen years ago I weighed 340 pounds and was a full-blown alcoholic. I was a single parent with a high school diploma, three kids, and no future I could see for myself. At that crucial point in my life I had the great fortune to meet people who believed in me when I couldn't. Would you permit me to return the favor and believe in you?

Today, eighteen years in recovery, I am a psychologist with a Ph.D. I'm a pioneer in the field of eating disorders, I'm in seven Who's Who publications, a columnist for two counseling magazines, a director of the International Association of Eating Disorders Professionals, and have opened centers for the treatment of eating disorders across the country. But most important, I am happy. My life is rich and full. I have many deep and meaningful relationships. I no longer live in that despairing state of isolation I knew when I was active in my disease. I'm a success story, and you can be one, too.

There's a psychotherapeutic principle I believe in, that you can't take a patient where you haven't been yourself. Because I am an alcoholic as well as a food addict, I know the needs of both and how they differ, especially in the way they respond to treatment. I know addiction from the inside out, and I attribute the high rate of success in our treatment centers to my once having been in the same situation my patients are in. Cross-addiction is more common than most people realize. Because so many alcoholics develop an addiction to food, especially sugar, while in recovery, it is beneficial to treat both addictions at once. "Substituting one addiction for another is like changing chairs on the *Titanic*." It's important addicts learn that early. Without that knowledge they may substitute one addiction for another. Addiction is addiction. There is not any one that is not life threatening.

Treatment at Janet Greeson's "Your Life Matters" consists of a ten- to twenty-eight-day program (length varies according to insurance coverage) of three nutritionally balanced low-fat meals a day; abstinence from sugar, caffeine, white flour, and other mood-altering substances; exercise of up to an hour each day; cognitive groups; intensive, action-oriented group therapy; learning and enactment of social skills; and nightly attendance at Overeaters Anonymous and other 12-Step programs. Much of this program can be replicated by reading this book and participating wholeheartedly in its activities.

My treatment philosophy in this book reflects the particular needs of the food addict. Nearly all food addicts come into treatment voluntarily, desperate for help, whereas many people admitted into drug and alcohol treatment centers are required to do so by the courts, employers, or other authorities. Alcohol and drug addicts have often built up a false and very tough ego structure that must be broken down before they can get better. Food addicts have been so humiliated by their disease they don't need to undergo the breaking down of ego structures. More likely, they come in with low self-esteem, which they fill up with food. They see themselves in terms of externals—the roles they play in life of spouse, parent, son, daughter, employee—and when they enter treatment and can't play those roles or stuff their emptiness with food, they are terribly vulnerable. We treat them gently. We make them feel safe, warm, and loved. In that protective environment, with their regular lives in suspension, they are often able to make miraculous and permanent transformations.

My own attitudes toward healing have been greatly influenced by Gerald G. Jampolsky, M.D., author of *Teach Only Love*. He writes, "Attitudinal healing recognizes a reality that is not connected to troubles, upsets, or even tragedies. That reality is love. Love is entered and assimilated only as our mind loses interest in either fighting against or succumbing to the miseries of life . . . The truth of love cannot be applied; it can only fill our hearts. Once this is done we will instinctively act in an appropriate way."

I have discovered this to be consistently true. It is the source of the miracles that happen at my treatment centers all the time. We focus on emotions, the internal emptiness, and the lack of boundaries, and all the rest follows. First the body responds to the new way it's being fueled, and then the mind follows—not the judgmental, cynical, chaotic conscious mind, but the imprisoned spirit of the addict that yearns to be free. It responds to the new messages it is receiving and starts rattling its prison bars. By *doing*, not *thinking*, the body will set it free. Do you feel resistance in yourself to reading these words? That's your disease stirring. Take it along with you into these pages. It will never leave you, but after you've released your spirit, you can arrest the disease and put *it* behind bars, one day at a time.

In order to give up something you have needed as desperately as your addiction, you must replace it with something else, for nature abhors a vacuum. If you don't want to be reading this with a Devil Dog in each hand by the second chapter, you must do more than think. Thinking has gotten you where you are now. Addicts of all kinds go in for magical thinking. They like to go to doctors who give them pills and tell them they're going to be okay. They can go into individual therapy and get stuck in the talking mode forever. But there is no magic to getting better. You have to *do* something. You have to change. How many people do you know who have been going to therapists twice a week for five, ten, fifteen, and even twenty years and are still miserable? I know the one-on-one process sometimes works. I also know it's not always the solution. You might gain some new awareness in years of therapy, but I don't know if insight is enough. Knowledge makes you smart, but it doesn't necessarily give you recovery.

My philosophy of treatment is radically different from what most centers offer. We're about change more than just dealing with awareness and pain. Because food addicts are isolates, we stress the development of intimacy skills. Other treatment centers focus on past issues, but I believe people are going to deal with their pain anyway, and if our therapists focus on it alone, the patients still leave with the problem of feeling isolated, incapable of intimacy, and not knowing how to really live. We teach and get them to practice the basic social skills they may have forgotten or, if they grew up in a dysfunctional family, they may never have learned, so they can achieve the intimacy they desire.

The only time we deal with the past is when patients have important unfinished business, hurts that are blocking them and need to be expressed, particularly anything that has been kept a secret, such as sexual or other forms of child abuse. "You're only as sick as your secrets," and they are always an impediment to recovery. In order to build a new foundation for life, they have to be revealed, forgiven, and disposed of. I have found the incidence of childhood sexual abuse among food addicts far greater than in the average population. In fact, the figure is so high it makes me wonder whether there's a "funny uncle" in nearly every food addict's family closet. I have come to the conclusion that many food addictions develop because food is the only mood-altering substance readily available to children, and when they use it to help them over a trauma, it becomes a lifelong coping mechanism. The use of food as a reducer of childhood stress is nearly universal. When babies cry, what happens? They get a bottle.

When a patient has unfinished business, we deal with it in psychodrama and group therapy. In psychodrama the incidences of physical and emotional abuse, loss, and guilt over a past event are redramatized so the feelings of anger and pain surrounding them can be identified and expressed. A lot of people have never experienced that pain because they were afraid nobody was going to be there for them. Sometimes the experience is overwhelming, and they're afraid they're going to lose control, but the pain of those traumatic events must be reexperienced before healing can take place. You can't go around it, deny it, or back away from it. The only way out is through the experience, with a therapist, a group, a buddy, or all three.

Patients go through the pain in a safe environment with people they trust, people they can count on to give them the support they need. People share secrets about their lives that no one else in the world knows. In the process their shared vulnerabilities bond them for life. Even if they don't carry on a relationship with each other physically, they remain bonded spiritually because they have assisted each other in a powerful healing process, a kind of emotional chemotherapy, exorcising destructive feelings they have been holding on to that have been making them ill all their lives.

Once they've identified their feelings, they need to learn to experience and express them to keep from exploding them in a binge or a purge. Addicts haven't learned how to trust their feelings or listen to their emotions. They haven't learned to take actions on their thoughts, not their feelings. A lot of addicted people don't even realize that feelings pass, that they don't have to own them forever.

Other than clearing up major issues of unfinished business, our psychotherapeutic approach is not to go back to day one to find out the root causes of behavior. There's not time for that. We focus on the feelings of here and now. Instead of concentrating on the behavior that the disease has caused, we work on creating new behavior, new identities, and new attitudes.

Too often people in therapy keep waiting for something to happen. I say you have to make it happen and get in touch with the energy that taking action releases. Then you can take that energy and go outside of yourself and feel a part of the universe, combining energies with others to create a sense of belonging. Knowing you're a part of something good and useful and making a contribution to it is what leads to recovery.

There's more resistance in the mind to getting well than there is in the body. Addicts have worked too hard for too many years reprogramming their minds to give it all up without a struggle, but if they don't think too much about what they need to do, they'll get there. The sickness that rages in food addicts' bodies is the direct result of what's going on in their heads, which are full of negative thoughts about themselves and others. Those thoughts are the bars that make up your prison. They need to be replaced with positive thoughts and action so the real you can be freed to have a life. Fortunately, the laws of physics are on our side: Everything in nature moves from a negative to a positive, but never the other way around. How many negative people attract you? Or do you gravitate toward those who feel good about themselves and others?

Changing negative thoughts to positive ones is called cognitive restructuring. For the mind to register a negative thought, it has to think it in a positive first. When it hears "Don't eat," the mind registers two sentences:

first, "Eat," and then, "Don't eat." I believe it's better to say "Stay sober and go to meetings" than the traditional "Don't drink and go to meetings," because the mind registers "Drink" before "Don't drink." Most people don't even realize that they have a choice about how they think and that knowledge is tremendously liberating. You can choose your thoughts but not your feelings. Feelings are reactions to thoughts.

There are only two things in life you can ever control: your thoughts and your behavior. You can't change your feelings; feelings just are. But you can change your response to them and then, like a miracle, the feelings will change without your doing anything about them. At the center we teach a "do-feel-believe" pattern of behavior change. Change the behavior whether you think it's going to work or not. **"Bring the body and the mind will follow." "Fake it till you make it."** These slogans (they will appear frequently in this book) are the distilled word-of-mouth wisdom repeated over and over by millions of people in 12-step programs who for many years have been successfully helping each other change their destructive behavior patterns. Nobody knows who said them first, but they're repeated like a litany because they work.

As you participate in the treatment section of this book, you will also be engaged in cognitive restructuring. Even while you sleep, your mind will be processing the change in thought patterns, and your dreams will be like road maps on the journey to recovery. Detours don't get you there. Belief systems simply cannot be penetrated in a weekend or even a week-long seminar, no matter how inspiring the lecturer or how confrontational the technique. In fact, highly confrontational seminars can do great damage, especially to food addicts, who tend to have a fragile ego structure. On the other hand, many of the more loving and supportive encounter groups that were popular in the sixties and seventies were on the right track, but they didn't give people the tools to change. They failed because they didn't go far enough.

HOW TO MAKE THE MOST OF THIS BOOK

At this point you are probably thinking, this is all very fine for people who can afford to go into treatment, but what about me? You can apply much of what is done in treatment at home. Here's how:

Section Two of this book is divided into twenty-eight days. For overeaters, there is a weight loss food plan and recipes designed to reorient your body to healthy eating, not take off a lot of pounds all at once, although you will definitely lose weight if you follow it. For bulimics and anorexics, there is a weight-maintenance and weight-gain food plan designed to reassure your body that you are now acting responsibly toward it.

Each day of the program includes a classroom lecture in which new concepts will be explained, followed by activities for you to complete. There will also be positive affirmations and meditations for you to practice. Sample journal entries appear at the end of each day of treatment describing what was seen, heard, felt, and learned by three typical patients, so you can identify with what might pertain to you. You will also be keeping your own journal to mark your progress through treatment. The twenty-eight days it takes to complete the program will be busy ones, and it will be necessary for you to find time to devote to it, for it will take your full involvement to leave the state of disease and enter the state of recovery.

You must read this book slowly—one day at a time for twenty-eight days—and participate 100 percent. If you read this book in two days, you cannot expect any results.

YOU CAN'T DO THIS ALONE!

If you have unfinished business of your own, particularly issues of childhood abuse, it will block your recovery, and I strongly urge you to seek therapy. Some mental health associations have a sliding-scale fee schedule, and you pay according to your income. On "Day Twenty-six" in the treatment section, I discuss "Choosing a Therapist." I suggest you read that section before you begin your search.

If you are fortunate not to have a lot of unfinished business in the way of your recovery, you still can't get there alone. Remember, food addiction is a disease of isolation. I highly recommend you follow the course of treatment with a buddy, someone you know who shares your problem, someone you feel close to and trust. It is also important to have someone to reach out to when the urge to act compulsively overwhelms you.

In addition, you will need to find 12-step meetings. Even if you follow the activities to the letter, you still need the power of a group. In the years I have been in recovery I have known hundreds of food addicts, many of whom had struggled unsuccessfully with their addiction all their lives, who worked the steps of the program and were released of their insane craving for food. Why it happens is a question I can't answer. How it works is one I can, for it is a well-defined process that involves only one thing: changing your behavior in a way that will make you happy, joyous, and free. The process is simple but not easy. The simple part is the lifting of the craving for food, which is unquestionably a blessing, but it is not easy to restore a life that has been damaged by addiction. The progress there is slow, hard work, but the saying "There are no failures in OA, only slow recovery" is one I have found to be true.

You may balk at the idea of needing to belong to a

group, but there's nothing to join. Twelve-step meetings require no membership, dues, or fees. They pass a basket at meetings to help meet the rent, but a voluntary contribution is the extent of the commitment anyone has to make.

Overeaters Anonymous groups are listed in most telephone directories, or you can call or write the national headquarters. Many lunch hour meetings take place in business districts; other meetings are held in the evenings in churches or schools. You may be surprised to find out you've been passing a meeting place regularly and didn't even know it was there.

When people first start going to meetings, I tell them to shop around. They are run by addicts like yourselves, so you are bound to meet some people who are too much to bear! Some meetings are more loving than others, and a few are too rigid or judgmental for comfort. "Take what you like and leave the rest." If the first group you find doesn't give you what you need, keep looking until you find one that does. Some meetings tend to focus on the addiction and others tend to focus on recovery. I prefer the latter. I know more than enough about my addiction but never enough about recovery. Once you find a group that makes you feel at home, keep going back. When patients ask me, "How long do I have to go to meetings?" I tell them, "Until you want to go." When you start out, it's good to know the feeling of "have to go" will leave, and you will want to go to the fellowship. We were not meant to live alone. Only the addict in you believes that, so it can continue to wield its power over you.

People who are born with endorphin deficiencies can become addicted to meetings, because being around loving, caring people raises their endorphin level. Their life is terrible, they feel awful, everything's going wrong, and someone suggests they go to a meeting. There they get an endorphin rush and immediately feel better, although they can't tell you exactly what was said or what happened to improve their mood. I wouldn't worry about becoming addicted to meetings, particularly if you're one of those born with an endorphin deficiency. To me, the benefits of the fellowship far outweigh any concern about whether people will become addicted to meetings because in themselves they fulfill a basic human need to be sociable.

You will probably find that after a few weeks of meetings, you will begin to crave them. Some people object to these 12-step programs as "just another addiction." My guess is that statement is either being made by a nonaddictive person or an addict in denial. Creating another craving to fill the void in the absence of food is essential until that void begins to be filled with the "real you."

You may also be one who objects to all the "God stuff," particularly if you were a victim of religious abuse in your childhood. The spirituality of a 12-step program has nothing to do with religion. If you are ready to accept the idea that your own power is not enough to cope with your addiction to food, you will soon discover that the power of the group is greater than your own. That can become the higher power you seek, and you need to go no further to find it. Once you identify with it, your own power is released. The experience is not mystical in any way. It's tangible. That is, it can be felt and needs no explanation or interpretation. After feeling bad for so long, even a few moments of this new joyfulness will keep you going until it grows. Just remember you're not responsible for the results. When you can let go of the outcome, I guarantee you it will turn out exactly as it's supposed to.

To me, spirituality is the positive energy you possess that has been blocked by your addiction. It is your own higher self. Instead of looking for some deity in the sky, I want you to go inside of yourself and get in touch with the good that lies within you. Did you ever see a baby you instantly liked? There are some babies I just don't take to, but then there are others whom I respond to with a smile because they are so completely in touch with the good within them. I like the baby even though it doesn't tell me I'm good-looking or nice or that it loves me. It's the baby's energy I'm experiencing, this joyous feeling of "there's absolutely nothing wrong with me." Babies can't tell you about it. You just sense it. It's as if they're saying, "Aren't I wonderful?" and of course they are, and you can feel the tremendous amount of energy behind that idea.

Or sometimes that energy is present in people who have died but whom you feel are still with you in some way—their spirit stays with you and continues to nurture you as the years go by because they have had such a positive impact on your life. That's the kind of spirit I mean: not an invisible authority figure but the positive and constructive force that lies in all of us like buried treasure beneath a slag heap of negative and destructive thoughts. As my good friend Father Leo Booth puts it, "You can take the alcohol out of the alcoholic, but you're still left with the 'ick.'" Transcending the "ick" is what spirituality is all about.

Recovery is about healthy rituals that bind us to others. It's being connected to the world in a meaningful way. It's also being connected to the Real You within, who has been imprisoned by addiction. The revelation of who that really is does not come about by learning something new but by the uncovering of who you are by nature. The bright colors of autumn are present in the leaves all along, but they can't be seen until the chlorophyll departs through their veins and returns to the tree. Your natural brilliance is like that. It's in you already, concealed by whatever defenses you have used all these years to protect your vulnerability. The unveiling of that hidden beauty is painful, like all change, but that pain is quickly forgotten when you see the spectacular results.

I am often amazed to discover how many food addicts don't see their own beauty. Debbie, an anorexic, was a particularly attractive patient who came into my office one day to talk about an episode of the television show *Beauty and the Beast*. As I listened to her, it became obvious to me that she identified more with the character of the Beast than the Beauty! The lovely, warm, ebullient woman who stood before me saw herself as ugly and an outcast. It became obvious to me that Debbie's obsession to transform what she saw as a completely unacceptable body image had led to her eating disorder.

I then recalled how struck I had been by a television interview with Ron Perlman, who plays the beast in *Beauty and the Beast*. He talked quite emotionally about how he related to his character because he was obese as a child. When asked what it was like to be in love, he responded, "The end of loneliness." Here was someone who had gone from being unacceptable to incredibly acceptable, still relating to other people with the pain of the outcast. When I saw *Phantom of the Opera*, I was struck by the way the main character was transformed from a grotesque figure into someone who moved me to tears by the end of the play. I have come to believe these and other dramatizations, such as *Mask* and *The Elephant Man*, all about people who have been ostracized because they do not meet the prescribed standard of physical beauty, strike a deep chord in us. Everyone can identify with their pain because none of us feels acceptable, even the beauties.

It's helpful to remember that even the fortunate ones, whose good looks we may envy, are rarely happy about their bodies. How tragic it is that we all seem to buy into the media myth that how we look is who we are! In the end, what does our outward appearance really mean? A package can be wrapped very attractively and expensively, but how long can anyone remain interested in an unopened gift? After that overrated first impression has been made, what people really relate to is your energy, and if there is nothing radiating from within that attracts others, you can be gift wrapped by Tiffany and it won't matter.

Getting real is what matters, the great relief of giving up all the false roles you thought you had to play to survive, to discover the joy of just being yourself and knowing it's all you need to be. Once you're real, you can be intimate with others. You can bond with them, and food will no longer be the focus of your life. Years ago if you had asked me who I was, I would have told you I was a housewife, a mother, a Brooklynite—I would have told you all different kinds of things about me or what I did, but all of them image. Today I would tell you I'm Janet, the caring person. The real me is loving and spontaneous and creative and attractive and sensual. I hope this book will help you reach beyond your image to find out who you really are. Most likely you don't even know who that is yet, but I can promise you, the person you've always wanted to be awaits you in recovery.

Not everyone has the courage to do what you're about to do, and I commend you for it. Be grateful for your pain, for it has gotten you this far. You're lucky. You're one of the chosen.

ACTIVITY: QUIZ

Are You a Food Addict?

You have an important choice to make. More important than what is happening around you is what is happening inside you. Answer the following questions honestly with a "yes" or "no."

1. Have you had a weight problem for
   longer than five years?   _____

2. Is there a history of obesity in your family? _____

3. Is there a history of depression or anxiety in your family? _____

4. Is there a history of alcoholism in your family? _____

5. Is there a history of drug abuse in your family? _____

6. Is food associated with good feelings in your family? _____

7. Does food make you feel good? _____

8. Do you ever get depressed about your weight? _____

9. Do you eat when you're not hungry? _____

10. Do you go on eating binges for no apparent reason? _____

11. Do you have difficulty concentrating or making decisions? _____

12. Do you plan secret binges? _____

13. Do you often feel sad, blue, irritable, or worried? _____

14. Do you ever have feelings of worthlessness? _____

15. Do you lack confidence in yourself? _____

16. Have you ever tried to lose weight by severely restricting your food intake? _____

17. Do you ever self-induce vomiting? _____

18. Do you often feel nervous and highstrung? _____

19. Have you ever lost interest or pleasure in usual activities, or have you had a decrease in your sex drive because of your weight? _____

20. Do you feel more tired than usual? _____

21. Have you wished yourself dead, attempted suicide, or feared dying? _____

22. Have you ever felt as if you didn't care anymore? _____

23. Do you feel depressed, guilty, or remorseful after overeating? _____

24. Do you become suddenly scared for no apparent reason? _____

25. Do you avoid or withdraw from others due to your weight or food intake? _____

26. Do you ever have spells of the blues, feel down in the dumps? _____

27. Are you experiencing sadness that doesn't seem to want to go away? _____

28. Do you see yourself as a loser at times? _____

29. Do you have difficulty asking for help? _____

30. Do you ever feel like nothing you do matters? _____

31. Have you ever lied about your weight? _____

32. Do little annoyances get on your nerves and irritate you? _____

33. Do you feel as if you won't be able to stop eating certain foods once you start? _____

34. Do you have an intense fear of getting fat? _____

35. Have you missed days of work because of overeating, weight, or related illness? _____

36. Do you take things very personally? _____

37. Do you overcommit yourself? _____

38. Do you feel responsible and think you are responsible for other people, or another person's feelings, thoughts, actions, choices, wants, needs, well-being, lack of well-being? _____

If you answered "yes" to ten or more of the questions, you have an important choice to make. You can choose a new life for yourself, free of food addiction and depression. You can stop living to eat and start eating to live.

2

Orientation to a New Life

If you follow the food plan, exercise between one half to one hour each day, attend at least three meetings of Overeaters Anonymous a week, and make a full commitment to yourself in the activities to change your mental attitude and behavior patterns, you will be a different person by the time you finish reading this book. It will be a gift to yourself that will keep on giving, and the next best thing to a treatment program.

FOOD PLAN

The food philosophy at Janet Greeson's "Your Life Matters" is simple: three high-fiber, low-fat meals a day, including foods from the four basic groups: meat, milk, and dairy; fruit; vegetables; and grain. Each of these food groups is represented at each meal to keep craving at a low level. One of the comments we hear most frequently from our patients is that the meals are satisfying. Because protein from red meat sources is hard on the kidneys and high in fat, the emphasis is on chicken and fish. Much research has been done on the connection between addiction and nutrition, and we have found that a high-protein diet, use of nutritional supplements, especially amino acids, and the elimination of all mood-altering substances, particularly white sugar and white flour, work best to help eliminate cravings as well as get the addict's body back in tune.

According to James Shanks, D.O., whose specialty is the field of addictionology, the body processes white flour molecularly, the same way as sugar. Refined sugars and white flour are linked to depression and mood swings, triggering the compulsion to binge in food addicts the same way alcohol does in the alcoholic. Refined sugars include honey, corn syrup, dextrose, and fructose. One expert I know calls these forms "sugar in drag." They have already been predigested, that is, broken down from a multiple to a single sugar molecule that is similar to the alcohol molecule. Complex sugars are present in fruit, vegetables, legumes, nuts, seeds, and whole grains, which provide all the carbohydrates you really need. They break down slowly in the digestive process and do not give the "rush" that triggers craving.

Binge foods are generally high in carbohydrates. Habitual bingeing releases large amounts of insulin, which stimulates the appetite ever further, prolonging the binge, and promotes the storage of the additional calories as fat. If you are a sweet binger, you can now understand why you can't stop after one; your body is conditioned to respond with a rush of insulin, resulting in uncontrollable hunger. In order to get your body to believe in you again, we take you off this cunning and powerful substance that has been acting like a drug in your system. Treating certain foods as mind-altering substances is the first step in real recovery for a food addict.

I recommend caffeine be eliminated because it, too, is a drug that separates mind from body, causing you to be in an altered state. Because it dilates the small blood vessels, they will contract during caffeine withdrawal, resulting in the headaches that are common during the first week of treatment. They will pass after a few days, as will the craving for caffeine. Substitute decaf coffee for a psychological lift, but don't apply this rigidly. Remember, rigidity is part of the addiction.

Pretty soon your body will begin to regulate itself without the need for artificial jolts of energy provided by these powerful and insidious drugs, sugar and caffeine. You will be amazed to discover how many of your mood swings, how much of your depression and anxiety has been caused by the habitual ingesting of these drugs.

Two food plans are presented in this program: one for people who want to lose weight, and the other for those who want to maintain or gain weight. The weight loss food plan is higher in protein so you won't feel so hungry between meals, with a lot of high-fiber vegetables and two servings of fruit a day. You may also have three servings of low-fat milk a day if you wish. A lot of people binge on grains, so we minimize them at first to avoid setting up cravings that will trigger one. Once your weight starts coming off, you can incorporate more grain into your food plan.

The calorie consumption per day for the weight loss menu is between 1,000 and 1,300 calories, depending on whether milk is being drunk. I don't recommend a food plan of less than a thousand calories a day because you're not likely to get the vitamins and minerals you need on less than that. I also recommend a multivitamin be taken each morning.

The average weight loss the first week is six to fifteen pounds. Most of that is usually water. Weight loss in the following weeks will usually be less dramatic, but it will be steady and mostly fat. How much weight people lose during treatment is not stressed (patients are weighed once a week, and I recommend you do the same), and the amount lost varies a great deal. I've seen people lose as much as thirty pounds and as little as four during the course of treatment. Remember that rapid weight loss may do wonders for your state of mind, but it's hardly ever permanent. We'd rather see you lose negative thoughts, pent-up anger, unexpressed grief, and harmful defense mechanisms during the twenty-eight days of treatment than a whole lot of weight. That will come off slowly and permanently in recovery.

Bulimics who don't need to lose weight and anorexics are put on a food plan of 1,800 or more calories a day to maintain or gain weight. It includes more grains, plus a list of cottage cheese, plain yogurt, green beans, chickpeas, baked fish, peanut butter, baked potato, brown rice, chunk tuna, and whole wheat bread. Anorexics also get high-protein snacks between meals of sandwiches, crackers and cheese, yogurt, and fruit. Contrary to the latest opinions by nutritional experts, our diabetic patients are refined-carbohydrate-sensitive and seem to do better on our food plan.

Weight gain for anorexics and bulimics is very small, if any. Their metabolism has been lowered because they've been surviving on so few calories. Their bodies have developed a famine mentality, take the additional calories, and turn them into fat to store for later use. It takes a while before structured exercise rebuilds their depleted muscle and organ tissue. People who resort to surgical intervention, such as having their stomachs tied or filled with a balloon, also undergo a change in basal metabolism. Lean body mass (muscle) is usually lost. Each time they lose fat, the body responds by holding on to the stores it has and cutting down on the amount of energy expended while increasing appetite. It's no wonder some anorexics complain of feeling fat—they do have a higher percentage of body fat.

Fasting causes a loss of protein in the form of lean body mass, and when anorexics and overeaters start to eat again after a fast, they fill up with fat, not protein and muscle. The only way to build up lean body mass after fasting is by exercise coupled with good nutrition.

Some physicians treating anorexics refrain from letting them exercise, but they really need to be exercising in order to build up their lean body mass.

We used to give the old-fashioned basal metabolism test using a face mask to determine how many calories a patient should be eating per day in order to lose or sustain weight, but this test is now done by a computer analysis called the Electroliprogram, and it is much more accurate than the old method. The test is remarkably simple. A device placed on the wrist for a mere fifteen seconds determines not only basal metabolism rate but also pounds and percentage of body fat, pounds and percentage of lean body mass, pounds and percentage of body water, and recommendations regarding loss of body fat.

And that's just the beginning! The computer then spews out a daily food plan with caloric recommendations based on the level and intensity of exercise the patient has selected. It breaks down each meal into kinds of proteins, carbohydrates, and fats that should be eaten and in what amount. It spells out fruits, vegetables, and grains that can be exchanged in making carbohydrate selections, and what kind of beverages may be used. It even gives an exercise prescription, complete with kind, duration, and calories burned for each day of the week.

These computer analyses are new, but because of their accuracy they are being adopted with great enthusiasm by many doctors, nutritionists, and treatment centers.

Twenty-eight days of regulated eating will result in a resumption of trust on the part of your body. It becomes convinced you're going to nourish it properly. Slow weight loss or gain, plus daily exercise, will actually raise your metabolism rate—as long as you don't skip meals. If you forsake breakfast and lunch, your body will once again stop trusting you and defend itself by craving food all night. Since your metabolism decreases about 10 percent when you sleep, nighttime is the worst possible time to be consuming extra calories.

Remember, if your metabolism rate is low, don't lose heart! You can increase it by eating three meals a day, exercising regularly, and losing weight gradually.

YOU'VE GOT TO MOVE THAT BODY

The exercise program at Janet Greeson's "Your Life Matters" is geared to the physical condition of the patient. We recommend aerobic exercise—large muscle, continuous motion in the form of walking, jogging, or running. People who are twenty to thirty pounds overweight exercise up to an hour each day by walking. That builds up stamina without causing them injury, which a more stressful form of exercise could do.

If you are not exercising regularly now, I'd like to get you into the habit of walking every day. It's a form of exercise that can be done anywhere and can be incorporated easily into a daily schedule of activity. Your goal should be to walk a minimum of twenty miles by the end of the twenty-eight days. The speed at which the patients in treatment walk is monitored by a nurse, taking regular pulse rates and educating them as to what a safe target pulse rate is for their age and weight. You can learn to monitor your own pulse rate.

Target heart rate is figured out by the following formula: 200 minus your age, multiplied by 60 percent, then divided by 6. That's how many heartbeats you should strive for in a ten-second period. Later, when you are more fit, you can increase your heart rate by multiplying by 70–85 percent. Four or five beats over your target means you should slow down. If you don't have a pedometer, you can gauge your distance: a mile is covered in a fifteen to twenty-five-minute fast-paced walk. It takes six weeks before you will really start to feel the benefits of daily exercise. Your body will become more shapely, you will feel less stressed, and your stamina will increase.

People who are not severely overweight can elect to jog, run, or take aerobics for their exercise period. At the center we have added a new form of exercise, dance, which the patients love—jazz, ethnic, and social dancing, even dirty dancing. Many overweight people have yearned to learn these dances but have been too intimidated by their size to join a dance class. Other forms of exercise we recommend are swimming (it slows down the burning of fat but it does burn the calories), the mini-trampoline, and rope skipping. Be sure you have good shoes if you choose the latter, to protect your Achilles tendons. The frequency recommended is four to seven days a week, every day if sedentary, beginning with twenty to thirty minutes and progressing to an hour. Intensity is determined by monitoring the pulse for your target rate.

Treadmills have the highest percentage of success of any exercise machine, that is, people will stay with the treadmill longer than any other machine. I think it's because they can do other activities while using it, such as reading or watching television.

In treatment we keep the exercise time to an hour because anything longer than that makes people hungry. It will also work off emotions that should be taken to group discussions.

GROUND RULES FOR CHANGE

Breaking Isolation

People who seek help for an eating disorder are often in advanced stages of isolation. Their relationship with food seems to be their only rewarding experience. The loneliness that is felt is so profound nothing can fill it up but a substance to numb the emptiness, and food addicts do such a thorough job of withdrawing from family and friends, they are convinced it is they who have been shut out by others. Their expertise in guessing how others feel and think about them and their obsession about rejection only enhance their isolation, making it difficult for them to reach out and ask for help.

When they come into treatment, they have often lost the ability to take the first step in communicating with others. Most of their conversations are light. People-pleasers have highly developed social skills in talking to others and are externally oriented. Their conversations are more listening than talking or mostly about other people. They remain on the surface of their ability to express themselves because they don't have the intimacy skills of sharing who they really are, what they're about, and what their needs are.

Then there are the isolates. Lacking the social skills of the people-pleasers or just too afraid to take the risk of rejection, they remain in their rooms where they read, watch television, or find other ways to be preoccupied so they can avoid having to communicate with their roommates. They don't want to be alone, even though they may say they do, and they are often desperately lonely. They, too, lack the skills to express who they really are.

But the people-pleasers are lonely, too. We find a feeling of emptiness prevails among them, a fear that they're not enough or as much of a person as they'd like to be.

One of the most important things we do is break that isolation by mandating contact with others. If patients consistently come back from their meetings and retire to their rooms to watch television, we will call them on their isolating behavior and tell them to start knocking on other people's doors. That simple act of taking the first step and asking the tentative "May I come in" is just as important as any insight they might have during a classroom lecture or therapy session, for they have taken an action and found out the real cause of their loneliness—themselves.

Another way we break the habit of isolation is by use of the buddy system. As soon as they enter treatment, new patients are given a buddy who takes them around the unit, shows them where everything is, explains the schedule, and in the process enriches his or her own recovery by reaching out to help others. No matter where patients go during treatment—for a walk, to the laundry, on a weekend pass—they go with a buddy. Lots of patients react intensely to the lack of privacy, but the truth is, being too private has allowed them to act self-destructively. We don't even let our patients cry in private. They've done too much of that already.

You can break out of the isolation you may be in at home by going to meetings of Overeaters Anonymous. There you will meet people who, like yourself, are willing to make profound changes to restore sanity in their lives. You may need more than an OA, however. You need a sponsor, and you may need a therapist. Overeaters Anonymous is a support group, not a therapy group, and the meetings are really not a place to go to seek therapy. Coping with an addiction in a group is a lot less painful than coping with it alone. I love the conference theme I used once: "We don't have it all together, but together we have it all." I have also noticed that people in 12-step meetings laugh a lot, not at jeering put-downs of others but at themselves. A room full of uproarious laughter is contagious and healing, and it takes the onus off recognizing you have an addiction. There are even those who come to see their addiction as a blessing, though it is not a requirement for membership in these wonderful fellowships. You can also break your isolation by reading this book with a buddy, with whom you are in constant contact. When you feel the need to reach out, your buddy will be there. When your buddy needs you, you'll be there, too. That kind of mutual support breeds self-respect.

Group Therapy

In treatment, ground rules for therapy are no gum chewing, smoking, or other distractions. Deal with the here and now, how you feel in the present moment. Speak for yourself in the first person, not of "you" or "we" but "I." Speak directly to an individual rather than to someone else about him or her. Be aware of the roles you play and your body messages. Be aware of how people in group remind you of other significant people in your life. Be an active listener. Expect periods of silence and confused feelings that may arise after a session is over. A simple contract is made: to be honest and chemically free, and to respect the confidentiality of the group. The same rules can apply to whatever group you choose to join during the twenty-eight days of this program, whether it is with a professional therapist or in an Anonymous meeting.

Ground rules for self-expression are very specific, for they clear the air of the smoke screen of nonfeelings and disbelief. Saying "I can't" is not allowed. It is a precondition of the mind, hardly ever of reality. It was once said that people couldn't go to the moon, couldn't fly, couldn't talk to each other over long distances through a wire, or see pictures on a box in their living room. "Can't" is a self-limiting thought that means you haven't come up with the right combination of actions to make it happen. "I can't" is corrected to "I won't."

"I don't know" is also not allowed. "I don't want to tell you" or "I don't believe in myself" or "I don't want to make the effort to find out" is what "I don't know" really means. "I'll try" is passive—aggressive. People don't change sitting on the fence. When that phrase is used in treatment, we say, "Trying is lying." "I should" is also forbidden, and anyone who uses it will be told to "Stop shoulding on yourself." The word "but" is also off limits. In a sentence, it negates anything that comes before it.

Exaggerating is a device used to get people to be truthful about what they say and the way they say it. Any time people say something in the victim mode, they're told to place the back of their hands dramatically on their foreheads. If they neglect to do so, others will provide the gesture for them.

At first it's frustrating to have so many restrictions put on the way you speak, but it eliminates the time-consuming, beating-around-the-bush babble that is allowed in more passive forms of therapy. There's no time for that in a treatment program. Many patients who have been in long-term therapy, especially one-on-one, are amazed to discover how much time and money they have wasted in self-indulgent verbalizing that never broke through their defenses to get to the heart of the matter—those explosive unexpressed feelings that lie behind layers of protective verbiage.

You can apply these ground rules for self-expression to your daily living, starting now. Be aware of how often you use the forbidden phrases. You will be amazed at how often others use them, too. Notice how they contribute to stuck thinking and cloudy communication. Try out your new way of expressing yourself in the safety of a 12-step meeting where honesty is encouraged and appreciated.

Within the small circle of eight to ten patients who meet with a counselor for group therapy four times a week, the most important work of treatment goes on, and the most intense bonding. People often come into treatment with no identity of their own. Once they get connected with a group, the other members help them see who they are and what they're doing. They first take on the identity of the group, and slowly out of that comes their own. People share things in a group they have told no one else in the world. Secrets, anger, grief, pain—much will be left behind in group therapy during the course of treatment, and these are of greater significance than any weight lost or gained during that time.

As a therapist, I pretty much ignore people when they first come into group because I can be pretty intimidating. People are very nervous in the beginning because they think I know their secrets. Some I do know from my own experience, and they can feel that. In the beginning they're too nervous to be addressed, and if I do, I might push them farther back into themselves, so I just let them watch what's happening with patients who have been there longer. If new people do open up the first day or two, they rarely get to the real problem but put on a performance instead, full of defenses and devoid of real feeling. I'm more interested in getting them to relate to something someone else is saying.

I watch the eyes of patients for "tele"—the transmission of trust—when they are so closely bonded to the group that they are lost in what's happening in the moment. This moment is when they know I wouldn't let anything harmful happen to them, and they are willing to experience fully what they need to share. Achieving that trust is my goal as a group therapist. Not everybody is capable of that kind of vulnerability, but for those who are, miracles can happen.

Hugging

Hugging can't be mandated, but it is an important part of treatment. Fat people generally don't get hugged a lot. Other people feel strange about hugging them, as if it were an intrusion. They sometimes perspire more than normal, they're not as sexually attractive as most people, and a lot of times are not sexually active either. Consequently, they develop touch deprivation or skin hunger, which they have learned to ignore.

I remember one time when my denial of skin hunger was broken through and nearly overwhelmed me. I was very overweight and hadn't been touched in a long time.

I went to see the movie *Fatso* with a date who was extremely skinny. When he put his arm around me I almost died. I was flooded with feelings and realized how long it had been since I had been touched.

At first, some patients are uncomfortable with all the hugging that goes on, but they're so sensitive to touch they quickly become aware they're not touching people either, and that's part of recovery. People need to be hugged in a nonthreatening, nonsexual, nurturing way, and the contact fosters intimacy and trust much more rapidly than words. It's an amazing Rx—fast, simple, free, and nonfattening.

I'll never forget Terry, a bulimic who came into treatment looking like a little old lady, although she was in her early twenties. Every Monday we have commencement, a ceremony for the patients who are leaving treatment that week. Terry arrived that day. She wouldn't talk to anyone and kept her head down, appearing almost psychotic, as if she had lost touch with reality. At the close of the ceremony everyone stood in a circle and held hands. Someone tried to hug her, and she angrily pulled her arm away. After the ceremony, I went up to where she had withdrawn into a corner, put my hand on her arm, and said, "You're going to be okay. The only choice you have to make is whether you're going to let me help you," and she started crying.

Her treatment was rocky. Terry had been sexually abused by her father and had a very disapproving mother. She never felt comfortable at home, never felt as if she fit in anywhere, and was not even comfortable inside her own skin. During treatment, transference took place with me, and I became the loving support she never had, giving her lots of encouragement. Today, she's a vibrant, beautiful woman who's honest, positive, and so real she just throws off this incredible, wonderful energy. There's a real sense of joy in her heart, and she's full of hugs for everyone. She's a lover. You can be one, too.

3

Food Plan and Recipes

In a treatment center, what patients eat is mandated. For the duration they are free of the nagging thoughts of what, when, and how much to eat. You may be thinking that doing this at home will be impossible because of your past dieting experiences, but this is not a diet, and no assumptions can be made at this point.

I'm convinced food addiction is different for everyone. The key is the "use" of food to negate, enhance, or stuff feelings. The food plan presented in the following pages is a guideline that will help you understand how to "use" food properly.

Prior to my own recovery, I was convinced that sugar was my only addictive substance. I went two years with the mentality "Lips that touch sugar will never touch mine," never recognizing that I was consuming three pounds of butter a week and the bread and potatoes to match.

Much research has been conducted at major medical centers during the past few years and the findings corroborate what I have believed for a long time—that excessive calories are not the cause of obesity, fat intake is. It's not a sweet tooth that gives people problems so much as a fat tooth!

I recommend the following amounts for each of the plans outlined here:

Weight Loss Plan: 15–20 percent fat
Weight Maintenance Plan: 30–35 percent fat
Weight Gain Plan: 45–50 percent fat

I recommend you limit your fat intake to 30 percent of the total calorie intake, at 9 calories per gram of fat. For instance, a 1,000-calorie limit would include 33 grams of fat. Although studies show that switching to a low-fat diet markedly increases the appetite for a few days, that ravenous period quickly passes. People who have lowered their fat intake in studies have not been found to compensate by eating more food.

Use one of the following three food plans to help you select your menus for the next twenty-eight days. Be sure to consult with your physician in order to tailor the plan to meet your individual health needs.

———————— WEIGHT-LOSS PLAN ————————

Breakfast	*Sample Menu*
1 milk/dairy	4 oz. cottage cheese
1 fruit	1 medium apple
2 starches/grains	1 slice whole wheat toast
	½ cup corn bran
1 protein/meat	16 oz. skim milk
1 fat	1 teaspoon margarine for toast
	Decaf coffee

Lunch	*Sample Menu*
2 vegetables	1 cup raw salad (2 vegetables)
1 starch/grain	1 tablespoon low-calorie dressing
1 protein/meat	4 oz. skinless chicken (baked or grilled)
	Water with lemon slice

Dinner	*Sample Menu*
2 vegetables	1 cup mixed vegetables
1 starch/grain	½ cup brown rice
1 protein/meat	3 oz. lean beef
	Decaf coffee

Nighttime Snack	*Sample Menu*
1 fruit or	8 oz. plain yogurt
1 milk/dairy	
½ cup sugar-free gelatin	½ cup sugar-free gelatin

—— WEIGHT-MAINTENANCE PLAN ——

Breakfast	*Sample Menu*
1 milk/dairy	8 oz. skim milk
2 fruits	½ cup pineapple chunks
	½ cup unsweetened cinnamon applesauce
2 starches/grains	1 slice whole wheat toast
	½ cup oatmeal
1 protein/meat	1 tablespoon peanut butter
1 fat	(= 1 protein/meat and 1 fat)
	Herbal tea

Lunch	*Sample Menu*
2 vegetables	½ cup sliced raw carrots
	½ broiled or raw medium tomato
2 starches/grains	2 slices whole wheat bread
2 proteins/meat	8 oz. tuna fish
1 fat	1 teaspoon mayonnaise
	Decaf iced tea

Dinner	*Sample Menu*
2 vegetables	1 cup raw salad
1 fruit	½ cup unsweetened mandarin oranges and sliced bananas
2 starches/grains	1 medium baked sweet potato
	½ cup cooked peas
1 protein/meat	3 oz. grilled pork chop
1 fat	1 tablespoon low-calorie dressing
1 milk/dairy	8 oz. skim milk
	Decaf coffee

Nighttime Snack	*Sample Menu*
1 fruit or	½ cup cantaloupe
1 milk/dairy	
½ cup sugar-free gelatin	½ cup sugar-free gelatin

WEIGHT-GAIN PLAN

Breakfast	*Sample Menu*
1 milk/dairy	8 oz. plain yogurt
2 fruits	½ small banana
	½ grapefruit
2 starches/grains	½ cup puffed rice
	1 slice whole wheat toast
1 protein/meat	16 oz. skim milk
1 fat	1 teaspoon margarine
	Decaf coffee

Lunch	*Sample Menu*
2 vegetables	1 cup raw cauliflower and carrots
2 fruits	4 tablespoons raisins
3 starches/grains	2 slices whole wheat bread
	2 rice cakes
2 proteins/meat	6 oz. lean roast beef
1 fat	1 teaspoon mayonnaise
	Decaf sugar-free soda

Dinner	*Sample Menu*
2 starches/grains	1 medium baked potato
	1 medium ear of corn
2 vegetables	1 cup steamed broccoli pieces
2 fats	4 oz. grated low-fat mozzarella cheese
1 protein/meat	4 oz. baked fish
2 fruits	¾ cup sliced strawberries
	½ cup sliced honeydew melon
1 milk/dairy	½ cup low-fat cottage cheese
	Herbal tea

Nighttime Snack	*Sample Menu*
1 fruit or	1 medium apple
1 milk/dairy	
½ cup sugar-free gelatin	½ cup sugar-free gelatin

RECOMMENDED FOOD LIST AND PORTION SIZES

PROTEIN

Meats

Red meat (lean beef, veal, lean pork, lamb)—3 oz.
Poultry (chicken, turkey, goose, capon, Cornish hen)—
    4 oz. (Remove skin before eating)
Fish and shellfish—4 oz. (Canned fish should be packed
    in water)

Dairy or nonmeat proteins

Eggs—2 medium
Dried beans, cooked—1 cup
Cottage cheese—4 oz. or ½ cup
Hard cheese—2 oz.
Low-fat plain yogurt—1 cup or 8 oz.
Tofu—4 oz.
Milk (skim or nonfat)—8 oz. (1 dairy or ½ protein
    portion)
Skim buttermilk—8 oz. (1 dairy or ½ protein portion)
Peanut butter (unsweetened)—1 tablespoon (add 1 fat)

VEGETABLES
½ cup

Alfalfa sprouts	Bean sprouts
Artichoke	Beans—dry
Asparagus	Beets
Bamboo shoots	Bok choy

Broccoli
Brussels sprouts
Cabbage
Carrots
Cauliflower
Celery
Chard
Chicory
Chinese cabbage
Collards
Cucumber
Dandelion greens
Eggplant
Endive
Escarole
Jicama
Kale
Lettuce
Mushrooms
Mustard greens
Okra
Onions

Parsley
Pepper—green/red
Pickles, dill
Pimientos
Radishes
Raw salad
Rhubarb
Rutabagas
Sauerkraut
Snow pea pods
Spinach
Squash (zucchini,
     summer, winter,
     yellow, spaghetti,
     etc.)
Tomatoes
Tomato juice, V-8
     (4 oz. = 1 portion)
Turnips
Watercress
Water chestnuts

FRUITS

Apple—1 medium
Apple juice—½ cup
Applesauce (sugar-free)—½ cup
Apricots (unsweetened)—3 medium
Banana—½ small
Berries—½ cup
Cantaloupe—½ cup
Casaba, Crenshaw—¼ melon
Cranberry juice (sugar-free)—1 cup

Fruit cocktail (sugar-free)—1 cup, not including the juice
Grapefruit—½
Honeydew—¼ melon
Lemons/limes—2
Nectarines—2 small or 1 large
Orange—1 medium/juice—1 cup
Peach—1
Pineapple—1 cup or ¼ pineapple
Plums—2
Prune juice—½ cup
Raisins (unsweetened)—2 tablespoons
Rhubarb—1 cup
Strawberries—¾ cup
Tangerines—2
Watermelon—1 cup

Avoid exotic fruits

Juice is a poor substitute for fresh fruit, and we suggest that you use it only when fresh fruit is unavailable. Buy fruit that is canned in juice, not corn syrup. Drain juice before eating.

STARCHES/GRAINS
½ cup unless stated otherwise

Barley, cooked
Beans—lima, navy, etc.
Bread—no white flour—1 slice
Buckwheat
Corn (no sugar)
    kernels—½ cup
    ear—1 medium
Corn bran

Grape-Nuts—no sugar
Grits, cooked
Groats, cooked
Kidney beans, cooked
Oat bran, cooked—4 teaspoons
Oatmeal, cooked
Parsnips—⅔ cup
Peas—dried (cooked)
Potato
    baked—1 medium
    mashed—½ cup
    sweet—1 small
Pumpkin—¾ cup
Rice—brown, puffed, 2 rice cakes
Shredded wheat
Wheat bran
Wheat germ—¼ cup
Yams

OILS, FATS
1 teaspoon unless otherwise indicated

Butter—be aware that it is an animal fat, which is high
    in cholesterol
Corn oil
Margarine (polyunsaturated only)
Olive oil
Safflower oil
Salad dressing—1 tablespoon (sugar must be the fifth
    listed ingredient or lower)
Sunflower oil
Vegetable oil

CONDIMENTS

—No more than 1 teaspoon per day of spices
—No more than 1 oz. per day of sauces

Bouillon (fat-free, low-salt)
Extracts (imitation, alcohol-free, such as vanilla)
Ketchup (sugar-free)
Lemon juice
Mayonnaise (low-calorie)
Mustard
Salsa
Salt substitute
Soy sauce (light, low-salt)
Spices and seasonings (sugar-free)
Tamari sauce (low-salt)
Vinegar
Worcestershire sauce

ITEMS TO BE AVOIDED AT ALL TIMES

Alcohol
Caffeine (coffee, tea, chocolate, soda, etc.)
Corn starch
Corn sweetener
Fried foods
Honey
Pasta containing white flour
Pizza made with white flour
Salt
Snack foods, including chips, pretzels, nuts
Sugar (dextrose, fructose, lactose, sucrose, glucose)
White flour

Any foods that can trigger a binge should be avoided.

FOOD PREPARATION

During the first stage of recovery, while your body is detoxifying from addictive substances, I recommend that you consider your kitchen a danger zone. Prepare the room by removing all triggering ingredients and prepared foods containing refined sugar and flour.

There are no dessert recipes in this section. It's difficult to make a dessert that serves just one, and I know too well that food addicts, once triggered, will eat something sweet until it's all gone. But no one goes overboard on the zests, the savories, the fresh herbs, piquants, and other flavorings that are featured in the recipes that follow.

As anyone who has tried to lose weight knows, nature hates a vacuum. Reduce portion size and the amount of fats, sugars, and salt you take into the body, and the mind obsesses on filling the void. My solution for the next twenty-eight days and beyond (but especially for the period of detoxification) is to substitute quality for quantity, with a focus on fresh flavors. Here's why:

One of the symptoms of depression is frozen feelings. We repress the ability to experience emotions, let alone emotional nuances, in exchange for the "peace" of feeling numb. The same is true for many overeaters. Like feelings, our ability to appreciate flavors has been numbed by excessive amounts of salt, sugar, and additives. Over time our taste buds lose the ability to distinguish the many nuances of flavor, but they can rapidly become resensitized on this food plan.

Into the void nature abhors comes an onrush of new flavors—not exotic, just fresh—and when they cross our newly sensitized taste buds, they create a biochemical effect on the brain. They fool it into thinking you are eating more because it is so busy processing all the new sensory data.

The key word is "fresh." Take nutmeg, for instance. If you rub a clove of nutmeg across a food grater, the powder you create is much more intensely flavorful than the kind you buy in a little tin that was grated long ago. The same can be said for many other "everyday" flavorings like garlic, ginger, and herbs: in their fresh form they are a symphony of flavor sensations that range from the subtle to the strong.

The focus on flavors will help you develop a new relationship to food, one defined by quality not quantity. The allowable fat per meal can be fragrant and fruity extra virgin olive oil, as well as boring old margarine. The sight of another filet of fish or skinless breast of chicken can cause you to burst into tears; the same food can also be redolent of fresh rosemary or a piquant tarragon sauce.

With the exception of some of the fresh herbs, everything on the following list of flavorings can be purchased at most supermarkets. Look in the gourmet section for items like imported mustard and extra virgin olive oil.

Flavorings

Garlic

Once you've experienced fresh minced garlic, you'll never be satisfied with using garlic powder—and no one needs the added salt. Garlic cloves are one of the most zestful and aromatic of flavorings as well as one of the most nutritionally beneficial. Garlic is essential to a good vinaigrette, and it creates an appetite for cooked vegetables like broccoli and squash. It is what makes a pesto potent. Buy heads of garlic with cloves that are firm to the touch. Elephant garlic is much milder than the smaller varieties.

Gingerroot

Powdered ginger is associated with desserts, but the freshly grated root is much more versatile and a new flavor experience. Prior to broiling, marinate fish in a paste of lemon zest and grated gingerroot Oriental style, or try the juice of the grated ginger mixed into fresh fruit. Gingerroot is peeled and then finely minced or grated. The root can also be sliced and boiled in water for a bracing hot tea.

Greens

Because the allowable cup of salad greens makes up the greater part of lunch or dinner, it should be as enjoyable as possible. Fortunately, salad greens come in a wide variety of flavors and textures, from buttery Boston lettuce to bitter radicchio and curly chicory. It's a good idea to mix the flavors. Arugula, sorrel, and watercress are strongly flavored and can be mixed with blander greens like Boston lettuce, spinach, iceberg, or romaine. Instead of predictable celery, try crisp slivers of endive or fennel with its hint of anisette. All these new flavors, together with the varying textures, combine to make the salad part of the meal much more than the usual grazing obligation.

Lemon

On a low-sodium diet, lemon saves the day. The tastebuds react to the sourness of the juice in a way that is similar to how they experience salt. The essence of the lemon's flavor is in its zest, the grated outer skin. Because it is a penetrating aromatic, it is excellent in marinades. You can also use it instead of vinegar in salad dressings.

Fresh Herbs

Fresh herbs can be bought in little plastic packets at the supermarket and specialty food stores, but they will never have the spark of flavor that the leaves release when picked fresh from the plant. Herbs are easy to cultivate, and in warm climates some grow like weeds. They are equally willing to grow in pots on a sunny windowsill. Because fresh herbs are so important to the twenty-eight-day flavor equation, I recommend that you go all out and buy your herbs as plants at a nursery or farmers' market. You can also order herb plants from seed catalogs. With your row of potted herbs growing on your windowsill, you can snip a few leaves or a sprig, as much or as little as you need, and the flavor and nutritional qualities will be at their peak (it is also very economical to grow your own).

The following herbs are usually used in their dried state, and their fresh flavor will be a new experience for many. Their aromatic qualities go a long way toward solving the problem most people have about allowable foods: blandness. Once you have tasted fresh rosemary on a baked potato, or a chicken breast stuffed with fresh tarragon, you can banish blandness forever.

BASIL A few leaves of this spicy, aromatic herb shredded into a bowl of bland-tasting greens will really wake up a salad. Add a half dozen chopped leaves during the last few minutes of cooking a tomato sauce, or serve with low-fat mozzarella sprinkled with olive oil.

MINT There are many varieties of fresh mint, the strongest being English peppermint. Milder are spearmint and the fruit-flavored mints like orange or apple. There's even a chocolate-flavored mint. Instead of dry mint, try a teaspoon of fresh-picked leaves in tabbouleh. Or snip a few leaves over sliced fresh fruit, stir, and let the mint permeate the fruit for an hour or two before serving. Fresh mint leaves are also a bracing pick-me-up. Just stuff the teapot with a cup of leaves, pour boiling water over them, and let them steep for twenty minutes. This tea is also delicious cold.

OREGANO Fresh oregano has a sharper, more pungent flavor than its dried form. Greek oregano is stronger than Italian. For either, small amounts go a long way to enhance the flavor of steamed vegetables, egg- and bean-based dishes, and tomato sauce. As with all fresh herbs, add during the last ten minutes of cooking.

ROSEMARY In its fresh form, this strongly aromatic herb with its piny undertones is much more adaptable in cookery than dried rosemary needles. The dark green leaves can be minced and sprinkled over a steamed or sauteed vegetable, or a sprig of it can be put into the cooking water of potatoes or other vegetables. A paste of crushed rosemary leaves and garlic rubbed over meat or fish prior to baking or broiling is an excellent flavor enhancer.

TARRAGON Tarragon loses its distinctive flavor when dried because the essence is in the oil. Fresh tarragon is a chicken breast's best friend. Try stuffing a few sprigs under the skin a few hours before broiling, then, before serving, remove along with the skin. The delicate perfume in the oil of the leaves will have been absorbed by the meat.

Sprigs of tarragon can also be stuffed into a bottle of white distilled vinegar to make a flavorful salad vinegar out of a very ordinary and economical product.

THYME Tiny peppery leaves of fresh thyme enhance all bean dishes, where they can be combined in equal parts with oregano and basil. Thyme also holds its flavor well in its dried form. Hang sprigs by their stems for a week, then put them whole into a small jar. Crush a few leaves right before using.

Nutmeg
Cloves of nutmeg, slightly smaller than pecans, are so much more flavorful freshly grated than in the powdered form. Try a sprinkling of nutmeg in a banana

yogurt or other fruit compote, or on any vegetable in the squash family. Nutmeg also flavors meat, marinades, and sauces.

Mushrooms

Portobello mushrooms are thick, meaty, and satisfying to chew. Sauteed in the allowed teaspoon of olive oil and sprinkled with herbs or mixed with a pesto, they are a meal of substance. Oyster mushrooms also have a meaty texture but are more delicate in flavor. As fresh mushrooms are so high in nutrients and low in fat and calories, they are well worth exploring beyond the usual snow-white variety we're accustomed to. There are many new mushrooms on the market, some that are eaten cooked, others raw. Try them and use the ones whose flavors and textures you like.

Mustard

Like champagne grapes, Dijon mustard grows in one small area of France. As mustard is one of the flavor mainstays of salad, you might as well treat yourself to a little jar of imported Dijon, particularly since it is likely to be free of added salt and other adulterants. Avoid most bright yellow prepared mustards, for they are full of both salt and sugar.

Olive Oil

That one teaspoon of fat allowed per meal can be in the form of extra virgin olive oil, for its fruity taste enhances both raw and cooked food. It is also nutritious and free of cholesterol. "Extra virgin" means from the first pressing of the olive, which produces the richest flavored oil. Choose oil that has a slightly greenish tinge and avoid those that are not cold pressed, for heat during the extraction process takes away some of the flavor as well as nutrients.

Thickeners

After blandness, the main problem with allowable foods is the lack of substance. Clear broth just doesn't do it. We yearn for our gravy. Purees are a flavorful form of soup, and an excellent alternative in preparing the allowable vegetables. Soup thickened with vegetable puree feels rich and hearty going down, and it lends variety to the ways these vegetables are usually eaten. For instance, try a "cream" soup of pumpkin, squash, broccoli, turnip, fennel, or cauliflower. Added to meat juices, the puree becomes a delicious gravy without using a drop of fat or any refined flour or cornstarch thickener.

Vegetable Puree

Puree of potato, carrot, leek, onion, turnip, or other root vegetables produces the best flavor in gravy. For soup, asparagus, broccoli, beans, beets, cabbage, carrots, fennel, cauliflower, leeks, celery, onions, rutabagas, spinach, squash, stringbeans, tomatoes, and turnips can all be pureed. Because these are not trigger foods, it is safe to make up a batch at a time and keep it in the refrigerator.

Wash, peel, and cut the vegetables into pieces. Cover root vegetables with cold water and cook until very tender. Save potato water, as it is a flavorful and nutritious thickener. Steam other vegetables until tender. Add a bouquet of fresh herbs in the last ten minutes of cooking and remove before mashing through a sieve or putting vegetable pieces through a food processor.

The puree can be served as a soup, or it can be used as a thickener for soup or stew. Spoon in the allowable amount of puree during the last few minutes of cooking.

To make gravy, deglaze a pan in which meat has been cooked by adding ½ cup low-sodium broth, simmering until all the bits of meat are dissolved and then stirring in ½ cup puree until blended.

Yogurt

Yogurt is a low-fat substitute for sour cream in dips, dressings, and sauces. In recipes it can also be substituted for buttermilk. Its cool and creamy blandness makes it an essential complement to the potency of the flavorings you will be using.

Cooking Techniques

Whenever possible, eat food raw. It minimizes the time spent in that danger zone, the kitchen. However, when it is necessary to cook the ingredients, try to use one of the following three flavor-enhancing methods:

Baking

Slow baking (at 325 to 350 degrees) using an uncovered pan or Dutch oven is the way to deepen the flavors of fruit, vegetables, and lean braised meat. Coat vegetables lightly with olive oil to promote browning and crispness. Onions slowly baked this way carmelize nicely. Deglaze the pan with water, add some mashed vegetable puree, and you have a flavorful gravy.

You can also braise in an open pan by adding water or low-sodium broth to the meat or vegetables. Tough, lean parts of meat become falling-apart tender by this process, while the slow baking at 325 degrees browns them, adding extra flavor. Additional low-fat broth can be added if the juices cook away. Add fresh herbs during the last 15 minutes of baking and cover.

Broiling

Marinating in a flavorful low-fat sauce tenderizes meat, fish, or chicken that is about to be broiled. Rinse off the marinade, brush the skinless piece of meat or fowl with olive oil, and broil it on a rack close to a fierce heat until it is well browned and just barely done in the middle. Broiling is preferred to frying because fat drains out of the meat while it broils, whereas fried meat cooks in its own fat.

Steaming

Steaming is the cooking process that best preserves the natural flavors and textures of the raw food; in addition, fewer nutrients are leached out into the cooking water during steaming than during boiling.

A good steamer with more than one layer is a staple of good eating. On one layer you can steam thin slices of the allowance of sweet potato or winter squash, and then add another tray of scallions, tofu, or other ingredients that cook quickly, toward the end of preparation. The steaming liquid can be saved for soups and sauces or for cooking root vegetables.

Sautéeing

Peanut oil can be heated to the smoky high heat needed for a quick stir-fry. Olive oil would burn at that temperature, but in its own range it is the preferred oil. To sautée, use a medium heat under the oil. Add minced garlic, onions, pepper, mushrooms, or other quick-cooking vegetables and stir to brown the ingredients evenly. When they are transparent and well browned, cover and let them continue to cook in their own steam; or add quicker-cooking ingredients with enough additional liquids to keep the contents from burning or sticking to the bottom of the pan.

Slow Cooking

Electric slow cookers are a great boon on a twenty-eight-day plan because they minimize time spent in the kitchen while getting the maximum benefit of the flavor of the food. In the morning prepare the ingredients, put them in the slow cooker, and add water. Eight to twelve hours later, the food's ready to be eaten with minimal time in the danger zone.

RECIPES

The following recipes can be followed for simple, high-quality eating, using ingredients described in the previous section. Portion size is based on the weight loss plan.

Salad Dressings

No prepared salad dressing can equal in flavor the one you make at home. Also you know it's free of salt and sugar and that the quality of the ingredients is the very best. The following recipes yield servings as indicated. Portion size is one tablespoon per serving unless otherwise indicated, which comprises the one allowable teaspoon of oil per meal.

MUSTARD VINAIGRETTE
(six servings)

> 2 tablespoons Dijon mustard
> 2 tablespoons lemon juice or tarragon vinegar
> 2 tablespoons extra virgin olive oil
> 1 clove garlic

Crush the garlic with the side of the knife to help release the oils that contain the essence of the flavoring. Then mince and put in a cereal bowl with the olive oil. Cover and let sit for at least 1 hour. Strain out the garlic before use, and save it for sautéeing.

Spoon the mustard into a small mixing bowl. Add the lemon juice or vinegar and stir until smooth. Add the oil a few drops at a time, using a wire whisk to incorporate it into the liquid until the mixture thickens. Sprinkle with freshly grated pepper.

CREAMY CUCUMBER DRESSING
(six servings)

> ½ cup cucumber, peeled and chopped coarsely
> 1 tablespoon fresh dill
> 1 large clove garlic
> zest of one lemon
> 1 tablespoon lemon juice or vinegar
> ¾ cup low-fat plain yogurt
> 1 tablespoon olive oil
> ½ teaspoon ground red pepper flakes
> ½ teaspoon ground cumin seed

Place the cucumber, dill, and garlic in the bowl of a food processor or blender and process until creamy. Pour into a bowl and mix with remaining ingredients. Because of the bulk of the cucumber and yogurt, this dressing yields 3 tablespoons per serving. Live it up!

RANCH DRESSING
(six servings—¾ cup low-fat yogurt)

> ½ package prepared ranch dressing mix
> 2 tablespoons lemon juice
> 2 tablespoons low-fat cottage cheese, mashed

Mix all the ingredients in a small bowl. Let the dressing sit for ½ hour before serving.

CAESAR SALAD DRESSING
(six servings)

The original salad dressing required a raw egg, but once you've tried this recipe you won't miss it at all. It is traditionally served over shredded romaine. Add the meal's bread allowance in the form of lightly toasted croutons.

2 tablespoons Dijon mustard
2 tablespoons lemon juice
2 tablespoons olive oil infused with garlic (see
   Mustard Vinaigrette, page 65)
1 teaspoon anchovy paste (avoid if you are
   restricting your sodium intake)
1 teaspoon Worcestershire sauce

Prepare the dressing as for Vinaigrette above. Add anchovy paste and Worcestershire sauce.

Sauces

These flavorful sauces are adapted from cuisines around the world, yet the ingredients are readily available, allowable foods from the regular food plan.

SATAY SAUCE
(two servings)

The coconut cream required for this fragrant Indonesian sauce can be found in most supermarkets, especially those that carry Spanish foods.

1 tablespoon peanut butter
1 clove finely minced garlic
1 teaspoon juice from freshly grated ginger
   root
2 teaspoons finely chopped scallions
1 tablespoon lime juice
½ teaspoon freshly ground coriander seeds
½ teaspoon freshly ground cumin
¼ teaspoon ground red pepper flakes
1 tablespoon canned unsweetened coconut
   cream

Combine all the ingredients in a blender or food processor. Blend until smooth. Spoon over meat, fish, or vegetables before serving.

YOGURT HORSERADISH SAUCE
(six servings)

This is a cold but fiery dip for raw vegetables, or a sauce for steamed vegetables or fish.

> 1 cup low-fat plain yogurt
> 1 cup grated fresh horseradish root, loosely packed

Stir the above ingredients together. Serve cold or at room temperature. Wow!

TOMATO SAUCE
(two servings)

> 1 pound fresh tomatoes, peeled and crushed; or,
> 1 1-pound can Italian plum tomatoes, whole or crushed
> 1 tablespoon olive oil
> 3 large cloves garlic, crushed and finely chopped
> ¼ cup onion, finely chopped
> ½ cup fresh brown mushrooms, sliced
> 1 tablespoon each fresh minced basil, oregano, and thyme
> freshly ground pepper to taste
> ½ cup grated hard cheese (low-salt Parmesan, one protein portion size)

Sautée the garlic and the onion in the olive oil until soft but not browned. Add the mushrooms and cook until they give up their liquid. Add the crushed tomatoes and simmer slowly in a covered heavy saucepan until the sauce becomes thick and smooth. Add the fresh herbs in the last 10 minutes of cooking. Sprinkle with grated cheese.

CURRY SAUCE
(three servings)

This can be used over meat or vegetables or can be the base of a stew. The flavors intensify if allowed to combine for several hours before serving. It's even better the next day.

> 1 tablespoon olive oil
> 1 small onion, chopped
> 1 teaspoon finely minced garlic
> 1 teaspoon minced peeled fresh gingerroot
> 1 teaspoon curry powder
> ½ cup carrots, peeled and sliced
> 1 cup chicken broth
> 1 bay leaf
> 1 teaspoon fresh or dried thyme
> grating of fresh pepper

In a saucepan slowly cook the onion, garlic, and gingerroot in the olive oil until soft. Add the rest of the ingredients and simmer, covered, for 30 minutes. Discard the bay leaf and puree by mashing or in a food processor.

PESTO
(four servings)

> 1 cup fresh basil leaves
> ½ cup fresh parsley leaves
> 3 cloves garlic, minced
> 4 tablespoons olive oil

> 2 tablespoons low-sodium Parmesan cheese
> 1 tablespoon low-sodium Romano cheese

Put the basil, parsley, and garlic in a food processor and pulse until blended. You can also use a blender, but be careful not to liquify the ingredients. Gradually add the oil a few drops at a time. Blend in the cheese. Store in the refrigerator until ready to use.

For a single ½-cup serving of whole wheat pasta, use 3 tablespoons of pesto. Before tossing the pesto with the spaghetti, dilute the pesto mixture with 1 tablespoon of the water the pasta has been cooking in. The same amount of pesto enhances the flavor of soups, purees, and any tomato-based sauce.

TANDOORI MARINADE
(four to six servings)

> 1 cup low-fat plain yogurt
> 2 cloves garlic, crushed and minced
> zest and juice of one lime
> ¼ cup grated gingerroot
> ½ teaspoon freshly ground cumin seeds
> ½ teaspoon freshly ground cardamom seeds
> ½ teaspoon freshly ground coriander seeds

Marinate meat for 6 hours. Before baking or broiling, remove from marinade and pat dry. Save the marinade in a jar in the refrigerator for future use.

FRUIT SAUCE
This sauce is a delicious alternative to eating a day's portion of two to four fruits.

> zest of 1 lemon
> ¼ cup fresh mint leaves
> 2 tablespoons raisins, prunes or other dried
>   fruit

*1–2 cups fresh fruit: a combination of any of
the recommended list of fruits. Be sure to
include a berry, such as strawberry,
raspberry, or blueberry.*
1 cup water
1 stick cinnamon

Cut the larger fruit into slices. Leave the berries
whole. Zest and slice the lemon. Simmer the fruit in the
water until the lemon slices are soft. Stir the bottom of
the pan frequently to prevent burning. Add the fresh
mint leaves. Remove cinnamon stick. Serve hot or cold,
or combine half and half with yogurt.

APPLE BUTTER
(one fruit)

There you are again staring down at yet another apple.
Here's an alternative: Cut it in quarters (leave the peel
and the core intact), put it into a saucepan with ½ cup
of water, cover and simmer until soft. Force the apple
through a food mill or a sieve. Discard the peel and
core. Pour the applesauce into a small baking pan, a
loaf pan, or a pie pan, and bake uncovered in a 350-
degree oven until the puree carmelizes. (Note: This
won't get brown in a microwave.) Stir the carmelized
pieces into the applesauce and keep baking and stirring
until the mixture turns thick and brown (about 30 minutes). Use this concentrated sweetness of pure apple
whenever you have a sugar craving. It is densely sweet
yet just your apple with its natural sugars intensified in
flavor by browning. One apple yields just enough butter
to prevent bingeing and yet satisfy that nagging craving
for sugar as you detoxify.

II

The Recovery Program

After 28 days of high-quality eating, I think you will find your body responding with a new kind of energy, as if it were an expensive car that had been previously running on a cheap form of gasoline and is now quietly, efficiently humming. Our precious bodies deserve to be fed high-quality food! The nourishment provided will then be equal to the quality of nourishment the following 28-day program will provide your mind and spirit.

4

Week One:
Nourishing the Spirit

You are in recovery once you take action. As soon as you make a decision to follow your food plan and do the activities at the end of each of the twenty-eight days, you are giving yourself something of value; you are "treating" yourself to a good life. Your recovery will consist of giving yourself the time each day to nourish your spirit, gain awareness, and experience a lessening of the true source of what's eating you. On days when time is short, it's important to do at least one activity, even if it's just a few lines in your diary. On a rainy weekend afternoon you may spend more time writing, thinking, meditating, and nourishing your spirit.

At the end of your first twenty-eight days of recovery, you will have worked through some major issues, your body will be cleansed of harmful substances, and your cravings for food will be put to rest. You will also have developed a new excitement about life, knowing who you really are.

For the first seven days of recovery you are still in the thrall of your body, that part of your being where your addiction lies. During this first week, as your body begins to respond to being treated as something of value, your mission is to nourish the mind as well, to value it and flood it with healing thoughts. You will begin to challenge the critical self-talk that creates a negative state of mind, that tells you change is not possible. The well-known "pink cloud" of early recovery is often the sudden and astonishing discovery that change *is* possible.

DAY ONE

Diary

Beginning today, keep a diary, not of your activities but of your thoughts, feelings, frustrations—what you say, learn, and come to understand—while working through the twenty-eight days. Make each entry as long or as short as you need, but write something every day. In this way you can measure your own progress and can make written commitments to yourself that are directed toward self-improvement. This diary will serve to strengthen your program of abstinence and recovery.

In order for this diary to serve any useful purpose in your life, it must be completed honestly and fearlessly. The entries are made by you, about you, and for you, and need to be shown to no one.

The act of writing helps us to formulate and clarify our thoughts, feelings, and observations. If you really work at this program, you are going to experience many changes and you need to write them down to process them. Writing also helps us to commit ourselves to our own consciousness unfolding. We are taking a step beyond simply thinking something when we make the effort to write it down. The more frequently you write, the easier it becomes, until one day you will sit down and the words will begin to flow out of the pen. Then what you write will become really valuable to your understanding, releasing the contents of your heart into your fingers, bypassing your head.

Because we cannot write down all our thoughts, we must choose the ones that are most important. In the process, we get more in touch with our sense of values. Writing is also a great stimulus to creativity. In writing down our conscious thoughts, useful associations and new ideas begin to emerge. Writing down the immediate thoughts makes more "room" for new avenues of thinking, new possibilities we may not have considered before.

In a psychological journal, writing can also serve as a harmless and effective technique for expressing feelings by giving us the opportunity to write about whatever powerful or disruptive emotion we may have bottled up inside us. The process of "letting off steam" through writing is one that many people have found extremely productive, for not only does it discharge tension, it also enables us to become aware of some of the underlying issues behind such tensions.

Drawings and other visual material can also be an important part of your journal. These may be images that come in the form of dreams, fantasies, or visualizations. Recording your dreams will increase your recall. You may want to keep your journal by your bedside so you can write them down immediately upon waking, while they are still fresh in your mind. The images evoked in dreams are often early clues to new changes and revelations about to occur in your conscious mind. The more you record them, the more access you will have to your dream life. Spontaneous drawings are also highly useful. These are made by putting pen to paper without any preconceived idea of what they will be like. The result can be of considerable value in self-understanding.

This diary is not a mere recording of facts, such as what you did with whom, or what you had for lunch. It is about feelings, particularly strong feelings, peak experiences, any "high" or "deep" feelings of peace, joy, love, expansion, awakening, and their circumstances and effects. Also include the negative feelings you have, and remember that strong negative reactions you have to other people may clarify your own unrecognized and projected problems.

Also record the techniques for change you are consciously using, and other unplanned experiences or situations that you find helpful in your ongoing growth process. This diary is also to be used as an honest recording of your personal weaknesses, character defects, and limitations that you want to be more aware of so you can work to change them. But give particular emphasis to the positive by including your successes—instances in which you did use the new tools you are learning to overcome the limitations. Include bright ideas that come to you, fantasies, stories, and situations that have special meaning to you and that may serve as seeds for further imaginative work. Record quotations you may have read or heard that are personally meaningful to you.

Use dialogue in your journal entries. We often find ourselves carrying on an imaginary conversation with a person or rehearsing an important event. Used consciously and deliberately, the inner dialogue can help us clarify our relationships to specific people, developing understanding and evoking insight. It is also possible to have a dialogue with things other than persons, for instance, with ideas and events. We can have a dialogue with the idea itself, or with a figure we construct that embodies the idea.

When we write out the dialogue rather than merely imagine it, we can reread it and study its content and meaning. One of the characteristics of these imaginary dialogues is they are more monologues than conversations. When we write down what we imagine the other person will say, his or her point of view may become clearer to us, and underlying motivations may reveal themselves to an extent that would not be possible in an unmonitored imaginary dialogue.

There is another form of dialogue that is helpful to write down, a simple and straightforward conversation with your own higher self. Within each of us is an endowment of wisdom, intuition, and a sense of purpose that can become a source of guidance in everyday life once we acknowledge its presence and validate its opinion. Trust the assumption that it is there, and it will answer you.

A final word: Trust the process of keeping a daily diary. It is a bridge from where you were to where you are and where you hope to be.

ACTIVITIES FOR DAY ONE

Assignment One: Diary, Day One

In your diary, answer the following questions:
—What do you hope to gain for yourself during this twenty-eight day program?
—What are your fears about changing?

Assignment Two: Affirmation
I Am a Celebration of Life

> I am not my body.
> I am free.
> I am as God created me.

Write the above affirmation from the book *A Course in Miracles* by Tara Singh in your diary and say it out loud every night before you go to bed. This affirmation addresses your spirit: the wonderful, disconnected, unseen part of you that is in the thrall of your addiction. It is your spirit that will give you the energy and positive outlook you need to change. Your spirit *is* the driving force of life. It makes life feel like a celebration.

"I am" statements are very important to people who habitually abuse themselves with negative self-talk. Addicts nearly always have this destructive internal voice that beats us up, especially when we are enjoying ourselves. This negative voice is toxic. It is trying to kill your spirit and it must be squashed. Affirmations are tools to assist you. It is not so much that affirmations drive out toxic thoughts, but that they create a positive environment that crowds out the negative energy attached to these thoughts.

Affirmations are healing messages to your spirit, which is being held hostage by your addiction but is yearning to be free, eager to change and grow and be light. Affirmations need to be said many times for them to take hold in the negative environment your addiction has created, and it takes time for these thoughts to feel real for you. You may first feel the change when you are less than fully conscious, like when you wake up in the morning. Suddenly you notice that the negative voice isn't so loud and incessant anymore. You may gradually become aware that you are less anxious, more peaceful, more willing to take risks. I can't explain how this happens, only that it does happen.

I know that for me God is the driving force in my life, but if you are troubled by the use of the word "God" in this affirmation or anywhere else in this book, find a substitute for that word that does not trouble you. Of if you can't find the right word, think of the letters as standing for "Good Orderly Direction." We can all use some of that!

A DAY IN THE LIFE

Martha I'm supposed to write about my feelings in this notebook every day, but I don't know when—

*what with all these medical tests, attending group all
morning and afternoon, plus special appointments with
this one and that one plus special group at night. I can't
believe the schedule, and I feel so tired I don't know if
I can last out the week.*

*Dear Diary: Here is a feeling. I am feeling scared
and mad. They don't want me to room by myself. I
tried to explain that all my life I have had my own
room, but their answer to that was, "Depression is
about isolation and we all feel better getting closer to
other people." That makes me scared. Scared and mad.
Let's see, what else does it say here to answer: "What
do you want for yourself here?" I just want to get better.
I hate my life and my body disgusts me. Please, God,
help me. I just want to be a good person.*

.

Martha came into treatment after several friends in
her recovery group in her home town near Seattle had
been to "Your Life Matters." Martha had belonged to
a support group of incest survivors for many years and
had been in therapy even longer. She stated that depression had really ruled most of her life. There would be
periods that lasted for weeks or months when Martha
would sink into deep depression. During those episodes
she would start eating as soon as she got up and eat
until she went to bed. These periodic depressions, with
their accompanying rapid weight gain, followed every
major loss of Martha's life, such as the death of her
father, who had deserted the family when she was in
her teens, and a bad falling-out with her brother and
his wife that lasted for two years. After each bout of
depression Martha managed to bounce back and return
to her active life, although the feeling of "gloom and
doom" never completely left her.

It was the loss of her teaching job at a small business
college, a victim of budget cuts, that triggered Martha's
worst period of depression. For two years she could
only find secretarial work, and during that time she

gradually began to see herself as an office temp ("The lowest of the low," she described it) instead of a professional. Then Martha's therapist became ill and gave up her practice, and that loss of someone she cared about pushed her over the edge.

DAY TWO

Step Study: Step One

Since Alcoholics Anonymous was formed in the 1930s, many forms of addiction—to food, people, work, sex, gambling, and other mood-altering drugs—have been recognized and treated by the 12-step program originally designed for alcoholism. Although food addicts and alcoholics respond differently to treatment programs, they both follow the Twelve Steps in recovery.

To get the most out of Step Study, buy or borrow a copy of *Alcoholics Anonymous* (the *Big Book*), published by Alcoholics Anonymous World Services, Inc. It's inexpensive and can be purchased at 12-step meeting places. The word "food" can be substituted for the word "alcohol" every time it appears in the text. The Twelve Steps are reprinted and adapted throughout with permission of Alcoholics Anonymous World Services, Inc. The AA original Twelve Steps are reprinted in their entirety at the end of this book. Read "The Doctor's Opinion" and Chapter One, "Bill's Story," in the *Big Book*.

THE FIRST STEP: "We admitted we were powerless over food—that our lives had become unmanageable."

Admitting powerlessness is a devastating thing. We are brought up to be competitive and believe that saying we can't win is a sign of weakness. Admitting powerlessness is an act of letting go, which is the opposite of the struggle we've been in for so long, a 180-degree turnaround in thought and action. The struggle has been one of mortal combat for our very souls, and it has been unceasing, a twenty-four-hour-a-day battle without respite, even in sleep. We can wake up in the middle of the night and not know why we're awake. We're not hungry, but our thoughts are on the contents of the refrigerator.

We are engaged in a struggle against the adversary that is "cunning, baffling, and powerful," that we can't see, can't really get in touch with, and the moment we let down our guard, it has a way of grabbing a new toehold, of pushing harder against us. Every time we think we know something about it, we find out we don't know anything at all, but we keep on trying to win.

As long as we keep up the struggle against the addiction we will lose, for we are only playing into its power. The struggle connects us with the addiction and it will always win, and the prize is our very lives. Our bodies are the battleground and we are stuck there, connected to our addiction and in its viselike grip, for as long as we continue to struggle. As soon as we surrender to our powerlessness, we are free to remove ourselves from the battleground and live like normal people—if not a normal, everyday life, at least one in which we are not constantly distracted by the need to struggle.

Let's look at the problem in retrospect. What has fighting won you so far? Take a look at what your success has been in beating this addiction your way. You may have had times when you seemed to be making progress, and then in a moment, as soon as you let down your guard—perhaps went to a wedding and had a tiny sliver of cake, or were feeling blue and bought yourself a treat—faster than you could say "Hostess Twinkies" the addiction had you back on your knees.

It's not your fault for being in the condition you are today. No amount of willpower can be used against an addiction that can't be outwitted or outmaneuvered.

If you still deny your problem has anything to do with being addicted and claim it is due to your inadequate self-will, remember that no one has more willpower over food than anorexics, and they lose the battle, too. Everyone loses as long as they continue to struggle, for an addiction that goes untreated gets progressively worse, never better.

Acceptance of powerlessness doesn't happen overnight. It moves through stages, from denial to anger to bargaining to depression and finally to surrender. It is a process you may already be in, experiencing all these feelings. That is a good sign; it means you are engaged in the process and beginning to give up the struggle.

After denial comes anger; who wants to have a chronic and incurable addiction? The trouble is, we addicts don't know how to express anger constructively and make it work for us. We are accustomed to venting anger in dysfunctional acting-out, usually by more compulsive eating. You may also experience scattershot anger—at everyone and everything, including this book. That's okay. Go for it. Anger is energy and needs to be discharged. Just don't express it in a way that harms yourself or others. Feelings of "It isn't fair!" and "What did I do to deserve this?" are legitimate but not helpful. You will move through them, so be patient with your state of mind and know it is part of the healing process.

Old angers may also emerge, over all the times you have been humiliated because of a condition you are beginning to realize is not your fault, over all the dances you didn't go to, the cliques that shunned you, the love affairs you didn't have. Honor these feelings. Don't try to numb or minimize them, no matter how much they hurt. They belong to you and need to be acknowledged.

After anger comes a renewal of denial: instead of struggling, you vow to negotiate with the addiction. You will follow a diet to the gram and will not snack in between meals. You will fast three days a week, eat normally three days, and binge on Sunday. You will enroll in a gym, go on a liquid protein diet, run three miles a day—all to no avail. The bargaining period is one last desperate attempt to live a "normal" life, and failure to conjure up the needed willpower will land you in the next phase of the surrender process: depression. Look at it as a gift. You are almost there.

You have lots of reasons to feel depressed. You are losing your best friend and constant companion: food. You are facing the prospect of having to change, and no one relishes that. Your future is uncertain. You are afraid. Acknowledge all these feelings, too. Denying them will only make you more depressed. Be good to yourself in this phase and begin to take the actions that will lead you to recovery—in spite of your state of mind.

Acceptance is the final phase of the process, and at first it will seem unnatural: Who cares to admit complete defeat? Practically no one, of course. Every natural instinct cries out against the idea of personal powerlessness. But believe me, the only way we can win is to surrender. When people balk at that idea, they forget they have already lost their will—to their addiction—for the progression of the addiction is a gradually diminished capability to exercise free will over use. Surrender is getting it back.

On page 448 of the *Big Book* a physician describes the phenomenon as follows: "After I had been around A.A. for seven months . . . I was finally able to say, 'Okay, God. It *is* true that I . . . really, really am a [food addict] of sorts. And it's all right with me. Now, what am I going to do about it?' When I stopped living in the problem and began living in the answer, the problem went away. From that moment on, I have not had a single compulsion to [overeat]."

When you finally stop fighting and loosen the desperate grip you hold on the addiction, the addiction inexplicably and miraculously loosens its desperate grip on you, and you can begin the journey of recovery. Surrender places the addict in you under house arrest, one day at a time. Remember, the person who got up the earliest this morning is the one with the longest sobriety. Every addict needs to surrender every day. It's the nature of the recovery process.

There are people who stop working the program at the point their compulsion is lifted. You may know alcoholics who quit drinking using the "white knuckle" approach, without working an Anonymous program. Although they were abstinent, their behavior remained the same. They didn't drink anymore, but they were still self-centered and egotistical and miserable most of the time, having denied themselves the one comfort they had found in life. Food addicts can also have abstinence without recovery. But recovery is about becoming "happy, joyous, and free." If you want that, too, you need to work on a 12-step program.

The admission of powerlessness must be complete. The text describes how in the early years of AA "none but the most desperate cases" could commit themselves to such a program. Those whose lives had not yet reached the point of utter unmanageability continued to believe that somehow, somewhere, someday, they were going to beat the addiction. They were destined to go through the addiction process to its final stages of living hell, at which time they would reach out for the program like "the drowning seize life preservers." That has changed today. Many people now come into 12-step programs before they've reached that bitter "low bottom" point.

The text warns that those who haven't hit bottom get introduced to the twelve steps and then decide to try more controlled eating: "When one [food addict] has planted in the mind of another the true nature of his malady, that person can never be the same again." You might go out and try using your best effort to control your eating just out of sheer rebellion and anger, but it will never be the same as it was. Your guilt will be twice as guilty, and your pain will be twice as painful. Before you read this book you probably didn't know there was an answer, or that the condition you're in is not your fault.

But once you understand the nature of the addiction and know how you can get better, if you go out and start participating in the addiction again, it's by conscious choice. When you know what you can do and won't do it, then you do become responsible for the condition you're in. You may still have to do it your way, and that's all right. Some food addicts have to get to the point of sheer hopelessness before they surrender. If you are one, just remember when you reach that point, you can resume your journey into recovery.

If you would like to save yourself the pain of testing your will against the disease of food addiction one more time, that, too, is your choice. If you have suffered enough, you can now let go of that deathlike grip on the end of your rope and after a few initial moments of panic, experience a joyful free-fall into sanity.

ACTIVITIES FOR DAY TWO

Assignment One: Your Case History

The story of Bill W., pages 1 through 16 in the *Big Book*, is a case history of addiction, covering a twelve- to fifteen-year period from the beginning to the final stages of the disease, and shows the progression of alcohol in Bill's life. Write a case history of your food addiction, showing how it has affected your life, drawing parallels to Bill W.'s story. Begin with the time in your life when food first became a problem and end it with where you are now and your hopes and plans for today.

Assignment Two: The Addictive Personality Profile

The following are characteristics of the addictive personality. Put a check by the ones with which you identify:

_____ Emotional extremes: You don't know anger, you know rage; you don't know fear, you know panic; you don't know pleasure, you know euphoria. With you it's all or nothing.

_____ Need for intensity: You relate to feelings, not facts; you crave excitement; you thrive on chaos.

_____ Need for immediate gratification: You want what you want when you want it and you want it now.

_____ Extreme thinking: You are either all wrong or you don't make mistakes. A situation is either black or white but never gray.

_____ Lack of identity: You need externals to feel alive. You must always be doing something, and you overidentify with whatever it is.

_____ Lack of boundaries: You don't know where you end and someone else begins.

_____ Lack of moderation: Whatever you do, you overdo. If something works, taking more of it will work better. You have a pattern of playing at cards for hours, or at sports until you drop from exhaustion.

_____ Overreaction: You overreact to things outside of you and underreact to things inside of you.

_____ People pleasing: You are always looking for approval from others because you can't give it to yourself.

_____ Perfectionism: If you can't do it perfectly, you won't do it at all.

_____ Inability to express feelings: Most of the time you feel numb.

_____ Low self-esteem: You never feel you're good enough.

_____ Attraction to pain: You are compelled to seek out potentially harmful situations and company.

_____ Assumption: You make assumptions about what others feel rather than ask, then act as if that feeling is real.

_____ Projection: You fantasize about what will happen and are surprised when it doesn't turn out the way you imagined.

_____ Isolation: You feel as if you don't belong anywhere.

_____ Judgmental attitude: You are constantly judging and defending both yourself and others.

_____ Need for excitement: If you create enough chaos in your life, you don't have to look at what's really going on.

_____ Poor impulse control: Once you get an idea in your head, you can't rest until you act on it; once you start something, you can't stop until it's finished.

_____ Poverty mentality: You worry there won't be enough of what you crave.

_____ Supersensitivity: All your life people have told you that you are too sensitive, that you over-react to things.

A DAY IN THE LIFE

Chuck   *The question is, "What events precipitated my coming here." As I think them over, I would sum it all up by saying loss. During the last nine months my life started to spiral downhill. My middle son took an overseas job, and his wife had their first baby in Saudi Arabia. Then my oldest son left his wife. Their two little ones came home to Grandpa and Grandma for a week and were angry, confused, crying. It was not a happy time, and I really care about my daughter-in-law and miss her company. Then my youngest child graduated from college and moved into her fiancé's apartment in Atlanta. My wife turned her empty room into a sewing room, crying the whole time, overwhelmed with her own grief. It was like I lost her, too.*

The song has many verses, and I might as well sing them all: My daughter's wedding was in September and I gave her away, another loss. Thanksgiving was a bust; instead of our three kids and their spouses and the grandchildren around our table, they were all sitting around other tables. My wife and I didn't prepare ourselves for what it would be like to sit there—just the two of us and that big turkey. Christmas was another loss. We decided we'd avoid the "home alone" approach and went to Atlanta to spend Christmas with the newlyweds. A big mistake. Instead of Christmas being the grand production we had put on every year for thirty-five years, it was a complete downer. The kids didn't have it together. We drove home Christmas Day with real bad feelings.

The thing that started the depression on one last downward spiral was when my wife went back to work. I'm semiretired now for three years. There I was, all alone in the house, just me, the dogs, the cats, and the refrigerator. I started eating a lot and couldn't stop because my depression had spiraled real bad. It got to the point where I couldn't sleep. In order not to disturb my wife I watched TV all night, clicking the remote until I could find something boring enough to put me to sleep. I clicked to a program where someone was talking about depression, food, and trauma. And here I am.

What do I want? Simple. I want this depression to go away. I want to take care of myself better, to make my wife happy. I want a good life for the two of us. By golly, we've earned it.

•

Chuck is fifty-five years old and works part-time at home as a telephone salesman. The oldest child of parents who both drank and did drugs, Chuck is a natural caregiver. He describes his relationship with his wife of thirty-eight years as "flaming codependents but really good friends." As long as Chuck and his wife had children and grandchildren around to nurture and care for, they were basically content with their lives. As a social worker, his wife has a continuing outlet for her caregiving needs, but now Chuck has only himself, the one person in his life whom he has continuously neglected.

Chuck came into treatment deeply into the crisis of his life. Until then, his emotions had never been out of control except for infrequent verbal outbursts, and he had great difficulty with his feelings of helplessness. A perpetual optimist, he didn't know how to handle prolonged bad feelings, particularly when they lasted for month after month.

Since childhood, Chuck had been a living time bomb, but the ticking couldn't even be heard because he was so focused on others. That time bomb ticking away was his repressed rage over his loss of childhood. But if anyone would have suggested during the first days of treatment that Chuck was an angry man, he would have brushed the comment aside with a joke.

The immediate goal for this patient was to chip away at his defenses, which still worked so well for him. By the second day, patients were seeking him out for comfort and advice. Chuck needed constant encouragement to focus on his own feelings and to nurture himself.

DAY THREE

Values, Attitudes, and Beliefs

You may be wondering how people can turn their lives around in twenty-eight days, especially when they may have spent a lifetime trying unsuccessfully to do just that! The answer is, you can't turn a life around unless you find a direction it's preferable to go in. Nature abhors a vacuum; one belief can't be removed without substituting another. In treatment we systematically replace destructive, negative thoughts and behavior with loving behavior—that is, such that will be constructive, productive, and additive in your life, and will increase your self-esteem and your self-worth.

How long you have held food as a value can help us make the distinction as to who needs treatment. There is a timetable for behavior change, depending upon the duration of the behavior that needs to be changed. A *value*, something you hold for what it is, or for its own sake, is developed in one to five years of experience. Changing a value takes ten to fifteen hours of instruction and equal commitment.

An *attitude* is a viewpoint that you have that you really need your substance of choice to exist. It involves your physical, mental, emotional, and spiritual habits, and it is difficult to change. It is the value you hold for food plus time, between five to ten years of experience. Changing an attitude takes twenty to thirty-six hours of instruction and equal commitment.

A *belief* is a strongly held commitment developed over time through the integration of values and attitudes. If you've held food as an important integral part of your life for more than ten years, or have been using food to cope with life for more than ten years, your belief will require at least thirty days to change. You have spent a long time in a relationship with food instead of people and need to change some deeply held convictions about yourself. You will be working through this section of the book on faith. I commend you for that and encourage you to keep slogging on even when you are convinced you will fail. Remember the timetable. It can't be shortened but it *does work*.

If you have always isolated yourself from your feelings, you probably have a big problem in trusting others and believe you are basically unlovable. That deeply held belief is particularly difficult to change, impossible without a loving and nurturing environment. But it can be changed, and frequently is at Janet Greeson's "Your Life Matters." When people come into treatment who don't know how to be a social being, we teach them how. We love them until they can love themselves. This kind of change takes place not just with the help of the staff, but with the others in treatment, for they quickly learn that healing takes place when they give to others, and that giving back is what nudges out the old behavior. Often the people who come in the most shut down are the ones who become the most responsive to the loneliness and awkward feelings of the newcomer. Within two or three weeks they begin giving back in full measure the gift they have just received.

The process of behavior change consists of DO, FEEL, and BELIEVE. You can think until you disappear into your navel. You've got to *act*. Think of all the self-help books you have read that had only momentary effect on your life. That's because your participation was passive. "You can't think your way into good action, but you can act your way into good thinking." The best way to increase your self-esteem is to do "esteemable" things!

Behavior precedes feeling: you don't hurt until you stub your toe. If you take an action, even if you don't understand why you're doing it and have no idea what's going to happen, afterward you will feel something—either better or worse. As a result of that feeling your attitude will shift one way or another, and after enough shift in attitude, your belief will follow.

In the twenty-eight days of treatment, you will be doing a lot of things that you don't understand, until one day you notice a change in the way you feel. At that point, you won't need to examine why these actions work or even how they work, for you'll know they do work. Food addiction is a disease about feelings. Because they're part of the problem, they're also part of the solution. They are the way in and the way out. You will know you are working at this program when you feel it working in you.

ACTIVITIES FOR DAY THREE

Assignment One: Value, Attitude, Belief Clarification Chart

Divide a sheet of paper into three columns and label the columns "Value," "Attitude," and "Belief." The first column will be for things, people, and activities—whatever you have put a value on for less than five years. The second column is for things you have valued for the past five to ten years, and the third for things you have valued for longer than ten years.

For example, let's say you chose three things you have valued for less than five years: (1) motorcycle riding, (2) Saturday dinners with the neighbors, and (3) working for yourself. For each, describe (1) whether you do it alone or with others, (2) whether your mother and/or father valued it, (3) whether you want people you love to value it, (4) whether eating is involved, and (5) the last time you did it.

By the time your chart is finished, you will get a good clarification of what kinds of value you give things in your life, and whether you are consistent or changing in what you value. Consider the values you now have and think ahead to five years from now. Would you like them to be the same or different in the future? If the same, how can you enrich them further? If different, how can they be replaced with something better?

Assignment Two: Changing Values

What changes would you like to make—in your values, your attitudes, your beliefs, your life-style—whatever you see going on in your life that is keeping you from being happy? Make a list.

Assignment Three: Nourishing the Real You

Deep down, most of us know who we really are. The problem is a lack of energy, an inability to actualize our being. We all have secret desires and dreams about being or doing something, but we don't seem to have the energy to fulfill those dreams. But we *do* have the energy within us, it is merely dormant and needs to be enticed and expanded so the real person you are can take meaningful action.

Take as an example a person who longs to play the guitar well. The instrument sits in its case in a corner, and year after year goes by without this musically gifted person mastering even the basics of playing it. There is no energy around following his deepest desires, no matter how much he tries to pep-talk himself into picking up the guitar and learning.

But once the energy that is lying dormant has been ignited, there will be no need for pep talks or other motivation techniques. The guitar will be taken up like an old friend and played many times a day, even if just for a few minutes. The desire to make the pleasurable activity a regular part of one's life is "suddenly" there.

This exercise is designed to be an energy enticer for helping you do whatever it is that gives you pleasure.

1. Write down the sentence, "The child I am is glad to see you." Close your eyes for a moment and see in your mind a child of two or three who is glad to see someone—running with arms outstretched, screaming with glee, jumping up and down.

Write down the names of three people you were glad to see as a child. Describe how glad you were to see them, and how just the sight of them filled you with joy. Now write the names of three people you are glad to see today. What is it about each one that makes you so glad? Do you let them know how glad they make you feel? If not, how could you let them know, if not with words, with gestures or a kind deed?

2. As quickly as you can, taking little time to think about the question, write down the words, "The child in me was glad to—" and complete the sentence with three activities you loved to do as a child. Maybe you had a passion for stringing beads, gluing matchstick towers together, sledding down a hill.

3. Write the words, "The child in me today is glad to—" and quickly complete with three or more things you love today with the same kind of passion—singing doo-wop, dancing the tango, going on the rides at water theme parks. Describe how doing these things makes you feel.

Assignment Four: Prime Time

Think about the days of the week. Which one is the most pleasurable for you? Now zero in on the most pleasurable time of that day. Do you feel the pull of its energy? Describe what you usually do during that favorite time of the week. Maybe it is Saturday morning when you can sleep a little later before running your errands. What else could you be doing with this, your best energy of the week? Take a look at your list from Part Three of the above exercise. Could one of them become a substitute for, say, going to the grocery store? What would happen if you used your best energy of the week doing one of your passions?

Assignment Three: You Are a Celebration of Life

Affirmation: Imagine Who You Are and Then Create Yourself.

What qualities do you want to possess in greater measure?

You are now going to compose a personalized affirmation to add to the short affirmation you memorized yesterday. Your personalized affirmation is made up of the statement "I am" followed by the qualities you listed above, and incorporating the changes you want to make. Remember, an affirmation is positive self-talk, what you say to yourself under your breath, by which you can replace those destructive negative messages you may be muttering to yourself all the time. Think of them as a cassette tape and your new messages as erasing the old.

For example, let's say you listed among the changes a desire to (1) lose forty pounds, (2) change professions, and (3) develop a better relationship with significant people in your life. In the qualities you want to possess you listed (1) self-confidence, (2) attractiveness, (3) success, and (4) serenity. To make your personal affirmation, you write:

"I am lovable. I am flexible and full of courage. I am fun to be with, and I care about others. I am attractive, successful, and serene. I am capable of achieving whatever goal I set for myself."

Don't wince. You *are* capable of being all these

things, and putting them in the present tense will make them happen. Your real self is yearning for this information and will readily begin to act on it, but that internal healer in you is also very literal. If you give it a command in the future tense, it will put off acting until the future. If you affirm that you are now what you want to become, it will begin at once to work for you. Remember "do, feel, believe." You won't feel and you won't believe until you do. Doing without belief is called faith. It *does* move mountains—by giving you a shovel and the will to do the job.

Make copies of this personalized affirmation and tape it to your refrigerator, post it above your desk, keep it at your bedside, and repeat it throughout the day, every day, throughout the week, until you begin to feel the results.

A DAY IN THE LIFE

Jenny   Well, I certainly had an interesting first day. I am assigned a roommate who didn't know she had a problem with people of color until, lo and behold, she's got to share a room with one. She made a real fuss. The reaction really surprised me. The other patients got so mad at her! It caused a big ruckus that ended with my potential roommate crying and asking me to forgive her. What surprised me most was how involved the other patients got, like they really cared. I guess it would normally take a person longer to find out if a place is for real, but Day One and I already know a lot about people here.

I know I'm supposed to write about my feelings in this booklet every day, and I will do that, but I just have to say that I'm very afraid of groups, and today really upset me deep down. I had a recent bad experience with a group that also gave out the image of trying to help people, but in the end, everyone just cared about themselves. Then I went on a weekend retreat that really did damage, like to my very soul. We were told our defenses had to be broken down, but that was just an excuse to humiliate people. I want to feel better, I want to stop hurting. I feel good about this place because of how they reacted to my roommate problem, but I'm very afraid of what might happen if I put my trust in a group again.

What I hope to gain from being here: I hope to stop obsessing about men. I want to stop apologizing for being me.

•

Jenny came into treatment at the age of twenty-eight, admitted for acute depression after breaking up with her married boyfriend—the second relationship with an unavailable man that had ended in pain. An additional blow came from a weekend retreat she had attended at the recommendation of her boss. He had said it would help her develop leadership skills. But there Jenny experienced severe damage to her already shaky self-esteem, causing her to retreat socially and lose enthusiasm for her job and being around other people. It was the death of her dog, however, that pushed her over the edge and made her seek help. She said, sobbing, that aside from food, her dog was the only thing in life she looked forward to seeing each day; the only real relationship she had.

Jenny came into the hospital neatly dressed, as if she were on a business appointment. She was a pleasant, soft-spoken, and attractive woman, but her tears would not stop flowing. That lack of control distressed her even more. She answered questions cautiously, as if there were a right and a wrong answer. However, she was extremely bright and hid behind the mask of her competence. An overachiever since her teens, Jenny held a Ph.D. in engineering and was working on an advanced degree in city planning. She approached treatment as another task, one which didn't involve her feelings at all.

DAY FOUR

Developing Self-Trust

"In food we trust, all others pay," is the motto of the food addict, but the lack of trust in others isn't the real problem. It's really ourselves that we can't trust. Developing self-trust is one of our most important tasks in recovery, and for many of us, one of the most difficult because we have failed ourselves so many times. We have gone on diet after diet, full of resolve and self-promises, only to fail each time to deliver on those promises. Or we have made attempts to change self-destructive behavior only to revert to our old ways when we are under stress or in a confrontational situation. No wonder we develop a lack of trust in ourselves. Over and over we fail to be our own best friend!

Developing self-trust comes from listening to that small voice within you that knows what is right for you. It's the voice that is drowned out by the constant negativity of our hypercritical inner addict who would tear us apart, while this little voice only wants to make us whole.

ACTIVITIES FOR DAY FOUR

Assignment One: The Agenda

Write in your journal quickly, without giving it much thought, some things you'd like to do. Write down as many as you can think of, with a minimum of ten. Then select five that you could start working toward now. They may involve saving money, learning something, or preparing for a change. There may be something on your list that you can just go out and do. Write these five things on a three-by-five index card and put it in a place where you will see it frequently. As you achieve the goals of your agenda, cross them off the list and replace them with other things on your list.

At all times, you will have five things you're working toward *for yourself.* This means you can make use of the time people usually "kill." You will always have energy around—that is, you feel motivated, excited, positive about—five things that keep your life interesting minute by minute, no matter where you are.

Keep adding to your list of things you want to do, and keep your agenda changing.

Assignment Two: "Chairman of the Board": A Guided Imagery

Lie comfortably and close your eyes. Begin by taking half a dozen slow, deep breaths. Imagine what your life would be like if your spirit, not your addiction, were in the driver's seat, taking you to your destiny. Now imagine your spirit sitting behind a big desk in charge of that life of yours. Imagine your spirit drawing up an agenda of five items, in order of priority—tasks that need to be done. Then observe how your spirit goes about tackling first one problem and then another. See how it draws upon resources, asks for help, tries new and daring approaches, and discards your tried and true methods, the ones you have invested so much in.

Now open your eyes. Thank your spirit for the guidance it has given you. Write down the five priorities. Choose one that you can do something about *today* to achieve and take an action. Tack the list of five priorities on your refrigerator door. Every time you take an action to assist you in achieving a priority, put a little check mark next to it.

Assignment Three: Developing Self-Trust

It's true, that small voice of the Real You *doesn't* often have reason to trust you, but you have all the reasons in the world to trust it. The following exercises are geared to engage that spirit in some meaningful dialogue and let it really occupy center stage for a while. By invoking that voice to come forward we strengthen it, and by becoming acquainted with this loyal internal companion, self-trust (and self-love) is nourished. In gratitude, our spirit begins to fill up our inner emptiness.

Using your right hand, write the following question: "Who am I?" Using your left hand, allow your spirit to write the answer. (If you are left-handed, do the reverse.)

Ask a second question: "Why am I here?" and allow your spirit to answer through your left hand.

Ask a third question: "What is standing in my way?" and allow your spirit to answer through your left hand.

Ask a fourth question: "What do I need?" and let your spirit answer.

Assignment Four: Affirmation: "I Am a Celebration of Life"

To the affirmation you have been saying to yourself upon retiring, add one more line. It will now read:

> "I am not my body. I am free.
> I am as God created me.
> I am safe and strong in
> My own company.
> I am not my body. I am free."

A DAY IN THE LIFE

Martha I have a terrible pounding headache at all times. They tell me it's sugar detox. It's the worst pain I have ever experienced. This program is not for me. Spent all of yesterday morning wasting valuable time talking about sex. What has that got to do with anything? I am going to start demanding more one-on-one therapy instead of all this group stuff. It's the only way I'm going to get better, and it's what I came here to do. I have to sit in a room with one other person and figure things out. But I can't do that either with this throbbing headache.

The afternoon group was taken up with the problem of trust. Trust? Who could I ever trust? It's such a strange word. I only think of it in terms of banks, like a trust account. That's the only trust I've ever known, and now I have no savings. I trusted getting a teaching degree because that would give me something to depend on. Nada. I couldn't trust my mother to protect me because I needed to be protected from her. I couldn't trust my father to protect me because he was a wimp. And then he packs his bags one day just before I was going to graduate from sixth grade and says, "I'll be back soon." He comes back when he's old and sick and needs me. So let's not talk about trust. I trusted my brother because we went through so much together and I protected him—I STOOD BETWEEN HIM AND MOM AND TOOK THE BLOWS—and he gets married, and he and his wife turn on me. So that's my story of trust. Please God or someone, help me. I am so miserable.

•

DAY FIVE

Frozen Feelings

Food addicts have learned to turn off their feelings, or bury them under layers of fat. Mostly what they feel is numb. My job is to get you to feel again, so you won't have to use food to medicate those emotions you haven't been able to handle any other way. Rather than deal with feelings that come from events that happened to you long ago, I want to focus on the feelings you have today, the results of events that are happening now. Maybe someone vented a lot of anger at you in an inappropriate way, or you were put down by a person you love. These are the feelings that are the most readily identifiable, and you need practice validating and expressing them in ways that make you feel competent about yourself. Competency has a lot to do with being able to tune in on what is happening to you in the moment, not trying to understand what happened to you long ago.

First, let's focus on identifying feelings. That may sound simplistic, but a lot of food addicts have denied their feelings so thoroughly they don't even know what they are anymore. They believe thinking is a feeling because they live in their heads. If you can substitute the words "I think" for "I feel," what you're describing is not a feeling. For example, "I feel this is an uplifting experience" is a judgment, not a feeling. However, if you can substitute "I am" for "I feel," you are in the realm of feelings. The words "I am lonely" and "I feel lonely" are one and the same. Simple adjectives and adverbs are required, not clauses preceded by "I feel that." You see how avoiding feelings is built right into the sentence structure of people who find them too threatening to express.

Feelings are most readily identified when they are a spontaneous response to something that happens in the present. Think of an occasion recently when someone said or did something that made you feel awful. Did you ignore those painful feelings, hoping they would go away, or tell yourself you must have done something to deserve it? The first thing to acknowledge is the fact that you have a feeling at all, and describe it to yourself, know that what you're experiencing is true to you. If your truth is questioned, be willing to bear the pain of someone else's not understanding. It's *you* who needs to validate your reality.

In the acknowledgment stage, it doesn't help a bit to analyze what's going on inside, deciding, "I feel this way because . . ." If someone walks over and stomps on your toe, your toe doesn't care if it was done on purpose or by accident! The first step of recovery is knowing your toe hurts! Why it hurts is not important. Nor is asking, is it all right for my toe to hurt? Or should it hurt this much? Or is it my fault that it hurts? Or what could I have done so that this wouldn't have happened? *Know* it hurts so you can take care of it! The obviousness of that acknowledgment is not at all simplistic. How many times has someone caused you pain and then said, "That didn't hurt" or "This hurts me a lot worse than it does you?" There are a lot of bullies in this world who use the tactic of denial to confuse people when they're in the midst of dealing with their pain. Analyzing it continues the short circuit. What's important is that *you* know you're in pain, and that's all the validation you need.

So there you are: Someone has just had an anger binge and dumped on you. You feel mixed up, scared, confused, angry, and depressed. In your mind you acknowledge your feelings. You skip "should," "ought," and "fault," and say, "Wow. I really feel mixed up, scared, confused, angry, and depressed." Notice you have *described* the experience to yourself, not *evaluated* it. If someone else does, and says something like, "You're not handling this very well" or "Don't worry. You'll be fine," you may want to respond, but stick to describing the experience: "Excuse me, I'd like to respond to that, but at the moment I'm overwhelmed." When you're out of control in a feeling, it's not the time to figure things out.

Sometimes people are pressed into making decisions in a distressed state because they don't realize they have the option *not* to respond when their feelings are out of control. They have the right to buy time by saying things like, "I don't know" or "I'll get back to you" or "I don't want to say right now." All these replies allow you time to process your feelings before taking action. Every time feelings of anger, confusion, or anxiety rise in you because people are bulldozing you, that is your cue to take care of your feelings, not to react to the prodding.

It's also not the time to get combative. If you respond to someone's temper tantrum by telling him he doesn't have a right to dump his anger on you, you get involved in a moral issue, which is bound to lead to an argument. You're not up to that right now, confused as you are in the midst of dealing with your pain. What would you do if the person were to angrily reply, "I don't get my rights from you. And furthermore..." The only rights you should focus on are your own rights, and the only person who is responsible for your own rights is you.

I heard a colleague of mine tell a story about a man who used to take out all his anger and frustration on Jewish people. One day he passed a rabbi on the street and made an ugly comment. The rabbi said, "Wait a minute."

"Yeah? What?" said the man.

"Is that all?" said the rabbi.

"No!"

"What else have you got to say?"

More garbage spewed forth. The rabbi kept asking "What else?" until the man had used up all the ugly things he could say. Then the rabbi said, "If I came over to your house and dumped all my garbage in your driveway, what would you do?"

The man said, "I'd have it hauled out. I don't need any of your garbage."

"That's right," said the rabbi, "and I'm leaving your garbage right here," and walked away.

Leaving the ugly words behind and walking away is a declaration of your rights, and a good choice in your state—you can't think and feel at the same time. When you declare your own rights, you have established an internal criterion that can't be taken away by someone else.

As you walk away, you can seek out a safe place to process your feelings. If you're in a situation where it's difficult to walk away, such as from an angry boss in an office, there's always a readily available and acceptable "safe place"—the bathroom. On your way, you can begin to reestablish your equilibrium by getting connected to your hurt feelings in a positive way. Are they connected to the fact that you care so much that you hurt? Are they connected to the fact that you have a very high sense of personal integrity and your life doesn't work well when you can't match it? Those are valuable attributes you have chosen to have. When you can't make sense of the big picture, you need to come back to the small part of the world that is you and say, "Okay, what can I do right now that would be useful, based on my values and who I am?" You need a reference, or you may enter into that state of free-floating anxiety that happens when people can't find one.

That state is common these days. We live in a world of relative values and uncertain morality. Everyone is struggling with these issues and no one seems to have the answers, lacking any kind of standardized frame of reference. Religious sources are supposed to offer a moral reference but often only add to the confusion. I heard about a woman who got terribly depressed because she had been listening to a tape that told her, "You'll know a person is a Christian by the fruits she's bearing," and she said, "But I'm not bearing any fruit. I must not be a Christian." I don't know much about that, but I know that orange trees don't bear fruit all year. What season was she in?

Free-floating anxiety is anxiety that doesn't have a reference, and it's likely to be the state you're in as you walk away from an unpleasant experience. You need some immediate orientation, starting with who you are right now, where you are, and what's true for you, and to forget about establishing references outside yourself. In your state, if you spend a lot of time trying to know more about what you're scared of before you get a reference, your free-floating anxiety can develop into stormy anxiety, a form of unintentional self-hypnosis, such as when you were a kid and spent the night together with other kids telling ghost stories. After a couple of hours you couldn't go to sleep!

Self-hypnosis is the loss of sensory awareness of the here and now. Anytime you're out of control, you're under self-hypnosis. You are in a stuck state and need to get unstuck. Unless you get out of it, your anxiety will trigger other negative responses, almost phobic in nature, vestigial memories of every other time in your life you've felt powerless and victimized; then you will start judging yourself for having the feelings in the first place. Words such as "stupid" and "dumb" and "how could you?" and images of other failures will soon have you immobilized.

If you lose yourself once more in the painful event, look at it as if it were a movie on your VCR and fast-forward it to the end. Then run it backward. If it were a war movie, it would start with the mushroom cloud and end with the uranium being put back in the mines. You can defuse the event in the same way. The terror of a traumatic event is the loss of self. If you can maintain orientation, you can deal with the problem and not the loss of power.

Remember, you are no longer doomed to remain in the stuck state that comes with denial of feelings. You have honored them and are now free to move out of that state into a competent one. Your first task is to ground yourself in the present moment. Become aware of stimuli that are not involved in your tension. A telephone rings, a horn honks outside your window, a baby cries. Orient yourself to the space you're in, feel what you're touching, observe what you're seeing. Be in the now so you aren't in every other situation that's made you feel this way, particularly the ones from your childhood when you were truly helpless. You're not that now. You're a competent adult, and you've got new tools to deal with these situations that used to make you so afraid.

Now that you are firmly grounded in the present, you need to reframe, not reblame. You need to ask yourself not the old question of "Whose fault is it?" but "What do I need?" Objectivity? Strength? Detachment? A relaxed state of mind? Flexibility and balance? Humor? When you have answered that question for yourself, ask another: "Where did I have that?" Put yourself into a situation where you had it and feel the power and the creativity of that moment. If you can't find a situation in which you were able to give yourself what you needed, visualize giving it to yourself now. Then run the sequence of the unpleasant event that just happened, freeze-frame, step into the scene, put your arms around yourself, and give yourself what you need. That's called reframing.

By using our feelings as a guide rather than a hindrance, we can learn to deal with the here and now. The origins of those feelings may never be discovered, and even if they are, they might not make any difference in how you cope with your present life. Merely acknowledging them and loving yourself for having them is a healthy beginning. The rest is practice.

ACTIVITIES FOR DAY FIVE

Assignment One: Emotional Inventory

Anger is but one feeling that food addicts have difficulty expressing. The following is a list of emotions that the normal person feels from time to time. As you read, you may be surprised that such a wide range and nuance of feeling is possible—and this is just a partial list! Rate each word based on the frequency with which you experience that emotion:

I feel this way: (1) Almost never; (2) Occasionally; (3) Often; (4) Almost constantly.

_____ Abandoned	_____ Attractive
_____ Accepted	_____ Bashful
_____ Accepting	_____ Beaten
_____ Affectionate	_____ Belittled
_____ Afraid	_____ Betrayed
_____ Agitated	_____ Bored
_____ Aggressive	_____ Brave
_____ Alienated	_____ Calm
_____ Angry	_____ Cheated
_____ Anxious	_____ Closed
_____ Appealing	_____ Comfortable
_____ Appreciated	_____ Committed
_____ Ashamed	_____ Compassionate
_____ Assertive	_____ Competent

____ Confident	____ Furious
____ Contemptuous	____ Giddy
____ Contented	____ Grateful
____ Courageous	____ Guilty
____ Creative	____ Happy
____ Critical	____ Hateful
____ Cruel	____ Homicidal
____ Curious	____ Hopeful
____ Debased	____ Hostile
____ Defeated	____ Humorous
____ Dependent	____ Hurt
____ Depressed	____ Ignored
____ Deprived	____ Immobilized
____ Determined	____ Impatient
____ Diminished	____ Important
____ Disappointed	____ Inadequate
____ Discouraged	____ Incompetent
____ Dispirited	____ Indecisive
____ Distant	____ Independent
____ Easygoing	____ Inferior
____ Embarrassed	____ Inhibited
____ Empathetic	____ Insane
____ Empty	____ Insecure
____ Energetic	____ Insulted
____ Enraged	____ Intimidated
____ Enthusiastic	____ Invaded
____ Envious	____ Involved
____ Excited	____ Jealous
____ Exhausted	____ Jovial
____ Extravagant	____ Lethargic
____ Fearful	____ Lighthearted
____ Friendly	____ Listless
____ Frisky	____ Lonely
____ Frustrated	____ Lovable

_____ Loved
_____ Loving
_____ Loyal
_____ Lustful
_____ Mad
_____ Manipulated
_____ Miserable
_____ Misunderstood
_____ Nervous
_____ Numb
_____ Nurturing
_____ Obligated
_____ Optimistic
_____ Panicky
_____ Passionate
_____ Peaceful
_____ Persecuted
_____ Pessimistic
_____ Playful
_____ Pleased
_____ Powerful
_____ Powerless
_____ Prejudiced
_____ Pressured
_____ Protective
_____ Proud
_____ Quiet
_____ Rejected
_____ Relaxed
_____ Repulsive
_____ Resentful
_____ Respected
_____ Restless
_____ Rewarded

_____ Sad
_____ Sadistic
_____ Scared
_____ Secure
_____ Sensual
_____ Sensuous
_____ Sexually abnormal
_____ Sexually aroused
_____ Sexy
_____ Shy
_____ Silly
_____ Sincere
_____ Sorry for myself
_____ Strong
_____ Stupid
_____ Submissive
_____ Suicidal
_____ Superior
_____ Supported
_____ Supportive
_____ Surprised
_____ Suspicious
_____ Sympathetic
_____ Tender
_____ Tense
_____ Terrified
_____ Thankful
_____ Threatened
_____ Timid
_____ Tired
_____ Tolerant
_____ Tormented
_____ Torn
_____ Trapped

_____ Trusting	_____ Upset
_____ Two-faced	_____ Vacant
_____ Unappreciated	_____ Valuable
_____ Unbelievable	_____ Weak
_____ Uncomfortable	_____ Weepy
_____ Understanding	_____ Worried
_____ Unhappy	_____ Youthful
_____ Unlovable	_____ Zestful
_____ Unworthy	

Assignment Two: Emotional Profile

Make a list of all the feelings you rated with a 4. This is your emotional profile, the state you are in most of the time. What does it tell you about the emotional climate you live in? How do you .want to change it? You *can* change how you feel. Sometimes it is the only thing that can be changed in a situation.

Draw a line through every feeling you would like to eliminate from the 4 category. Then go through the list and choose the feelings you want to use to describe yourself and add them to the list. Make an "I Am" affirmation for the next five days, using your list of "feeling" words.

Assignment Three: Learning to Feel Again

Life is about experiencing joy in the present moment, the only time when sensory experience can take place. It's a challenge to be in the here and now, especially for people who have numbed themselves in order to cope. By protecting themselves from the pain they also block off the joy. They spend their lives defending or protecting themselves but never experience complete joy.

The following activities will enable you to gradually build a tolerance to pleasure and body sensations. As you do them, remember:

—Stay aware in your body.

—If you find yourself spacing out, focus on breathing air in and out of your body.

"Lathering"

"Lather" is a good sensual word. You can almost feel its thickness and its smoothness. The next time you are washing your hands, take a few minutes and resensitize the experience by performing it with the eyes closed, slowing it down and being aware of all the details. Work up a good, rich lather and soap yourself all the way to your elbows. Feel the water when you rinse off the soap. Rub your skin well with a towel. Imagine how many of life's little pleasures go by unobserved and unappreciated by you every day.

Assignment Four: Song of the Shower

Awakening to small and ordinary sensory pleasures is one of the great joys of recovery. It means you don't have to do anything differently, just respond to what is already part of your life in a more heightened way. For instance, the morning shower can be something to rush through in order to get clean, or it can be a pleasurable body awakening through the skin, our largest sense organ. Sometimes we forget how luxurious it is to be able to stand under a warm-to-hot rush of water every morning! Not only does it awaken the sense organs, it charges the atmosphere with negative ions, producing the alpha state. Ever wonder why people sing or get their best ideas in the shower? They're responding to the charge of negative ions.

The exercise for today is to increase your attention to the entire showering experience. A bath, unfortunately, will not charge the atmosphere with negative ions. It will relax you but this activity is for stimulation. First, wet your body, head, hair and all, in water just approaching hot. Then, as your body temperature increases, turn up the water to just this side of hot and let it beat on your chest. This rush of warmth to your heart and the resulting increase in blood circulation will cause your body to feel as if it is opening up to warmth and well-being.

When you shampoo your hair, give your scalp a good massage with your fingertips. Then, while your conditioner is doing its work, scrub your body from head to foot with a fragrant soap that produces a lot of lather. Use a loofa or cactus fiber washcloth, something slightly abrasive that will stimulate all the nerve cells in your skin as well as the flow of blood in all your capillaries.

Now give your muscles a water massage, particularly the ones that are stressed. If you sit at a desk for a living, pay attention to your neck and shoulders. Let a vigorous jet of hot water massage that area, then follow the spine down to the lower back, another trouble area. Lean forward and let the water massage that area, then move so the jet of water goes up and down your spine. Don't forget your arms and legs.

Rinse your hair and body clean. This is usually the time for singing, for the warm moisture has opened all the passageways in the head. The song of the shower is usually on the hearty side. Often it is opera. It can be sung loud, for the acoustics are wonderful.

Once you're all rinsed off, shut off the hot water and turn on the cold full blast. Let the water revitalize you and awaken every part of your body. Stand under the water for a few minutes or simply for as long as you can bear it.

After the shower comes a vigorous towel rub, providing more stimulation, followed by the oils and moisturizers that keep the skin smooth and supple.

The morning shower may be a most ordinary and mundane activity, or it can be a daily celebration, a hymn of thanks to indoor plumbing, a ritual of awareness of life's small pleasures. Enjoying yourself doesn't have to be a big production. It can be as simple as a morning shower.

A DAY IN THE LIFE

Chuck *Today's group has really got me going. I'm feeling so much loss and sadness. The topic was family roles. I am the oldest and the scapegoat, the fat one. All I remember is that for many years my first name was Goddamnit and my middle name was Stupid, or sometimes it was the other way around. I was the placater and stepped in so my kid brother and sister wouldn't get hit by my parents. My weight became like a red flag to attract their attention. That way I became the focus of my parents' rage, especially in the case of my dad, who was violent. Part of my getting so big was about getting bigger than him. I remember, as a grown man, talking to my mom about all the beatings. She said, "Can't you remember all the times I would step in and whip you kids so your dad wouldn't?" She said it like she was really doing us some big favor. She couldn't acknowledge the fact that she hurt us.*

There's a lot of sadness and emptiness in me because I really feel deprived of the times when I was growing up when my dad and I could have been friends. A lot of loss there, and a lot of loss with my mom. But you know, there's something good even in things that are bad. Because of the way I was treated, I was determined not to repeat the abuse on my children. My brother has gone even further and says he won't have any children because there's something violent in our genes. That's pretty radical. The abuse stopped here as far as I'm concerned. I stopped it, but look what it's done to me. I want to make a change and don't know how to do it.

•

DAY SIX

What's Eating You Can Also Make You Sick!

The link between mental attitude and physical illness is finally being taken seriously by the medical establishment, and in the past decade a whole new field of study called psychoneuroimmunology, a combination of the fields of psychology and immunology, has emerged. During the 1980s, research conducted by the National Institute of Mental Health, New York's Mt. Sinai Hospital, and other major institutions has documented surprising new evidence that employment of the techniques used in this book to change a person's self-defeating state of mind—stress-reducing relaxation therapies, moderate physical exercise, visualization, cognitive restructuring, meditation, positive affirmations, and confronting traumatic memories—actually enhances the body's immune system. The new studies confirm what many already believed—that people who think sick are more likely to be sick, and that people who think well are more likely to be well.

The concept that emotions affect physical health has been around in medical circles for a long time. In the second century A.D., a Greek physician noted that unhappy women were more prone to develop cancer than happy women, and a belief that psychic imbalance (the four humors) caused disease was central to the practice of medicine in Europe until the rise of modern science in the seventeenth century. After that, however, the relationship between emotions and physical health was given as much credence among medical practitioners as the theories of witch doctors and faith healers. It is only in the last decade that we have seen a surprising turnaround in their thinking. Hundreds of studies have now been done that show that a person's state of mind affects the immune system.

These days, protecting your immune system is as important as getting a polio vaccination was in the 1950s, for our bodies' natural line of defense is under attack from many sources—AIDS and other viruses that attack the immune system, such as Epstein-Barr, herpes, and chronic fatigue syndrome, plus cancer, environmental contaminants, and high levels of stress.

In order to understand how we can help our immune system, we need to take a look at how that system works. It is a marvel of complexity, much of it still a mystery. A healthy immune system operates much like a well-disciplined army. The first line of defense is at the skin level. A wound or lesion will be surrounded by swarms of phagocytes, white blood cells that eat the invading bacterial cells until the phagocytes die in the process, forming the yellow-white substance commonly known as pus around the wound.

The secondary line of defense are the lymphocytes, such as B-cells, T-cells, and natural killer cells. They roam the bloodstream searching for antigens, foreign substances such as bacteria, viruses, or toxins. The lymphocytes then release antibodies, which destroy the invader.

Endorphins are the link between the immune system and the brain. They are neurotransmitters such as serotonin, acetylcholine, and norepinephrine, compounds that act like messengers shuttling electrical impulses between the nerve cells in the brain, triggering a highly complex response that begins in the hypothalamus and ends in the cells of the immune system. Recent discoveries have found that these neurotransmitters also play a role in controlling the autonomic nervous system, the part that operates automatically to regulate all the involuntary activity of the body. This connection between the autonomic nervous system and the immune system has caused the scientific community to completely rethink its position on how the body protects itself. The new research also shows that these messages can be communicated in both directions. Some of the neurotransmitters, such as the "feel good" opiate betaendorphin, originate in the immune system itself. In fact, these mood-altering transmitters have recently been found in all parts of the body, not just the brain! The idea of a feedback loop, that the central nervous system can influence the immune system, which can then influence the central nervous system, is creating much interest and excitement among researchers, and it further illustrates the biochemical linkages between body and mind.

Since the pioneering work of Dr. Hans Selye in the 1950s, hundreds of studies have been conducted that confirm his original research on the effects of emotional stress on the immune system, that neurotransmitters produced in the brain travel through the blood to alter the activity of the immune system on the cellular level. Not all stress is damaging. In fact, mild forms of stress can actually enhance the immune system, but unhealthy levels, particularly acute stress, can weaken it. Fear and rage, or inappropriate triggering of the fight-or-flight syndrome (which provided our ancestors with the adrenaline needed to escape from wild beasts but is of little help when confronting an angry spouse or boss), are the kinds of stress that do people harm. Unhealthy stress decreases the body's protein and fat synthesis and glucose use, diminishing the amount of insulin it produces. It also creates a biochemical domino effect that begins in the brain with an increase in the production of the hormone corticosterone, which in turn decreases the number of T-cells, B-cells, and natural killer cells, which patrol the immune system, destroying newly formed cancer cells and other invaders.

A major study conducted at New York's Mt. Sinai Hospital documented the impairment of the immune system in men whose wives had recently died. Their bereavement impaired the ability of their lymphocytes to destroy intruders. A study done there in 1984 on people hospitalized for depression documented a decline in the number of lymphocytes in their bloodstream.

Studies have also been done on the effects of alcohol on the immune system, and they convincingly show that it inhibits the response of the immune system's defense mechanisms, predisposing the heavy drinker to infection.

So far, the effects of positive mental states on the immune system have not been as well documented as the effects of negative mental states. In 1976, Norman Cousins's book describing how he overcame ankylosing spondylitis, a chronic, progressive disease of the spine, with vitamin C and laughter was interesting but anecdotal as far as the medical community was concerned. Bernie Siegel's books on the subject have helped millions. By the 1980s, hundreds of carefully controlled studies had found conclusive evidence that there is a strong link between mental attitude and physical health.

Stress reduction techniques have been found to lower blood pressure, the rate of respiration, and the triggering of the fight-or-flight response in the autonomic system, which other studies have found impairs the functioning of the immune system. Another study found that when subjects were hypnotized and given a suggestion that their white blood cells were like sharks devouring tiny fishlike antigens, the activity of their lymphocytes actually increased. Serotonin levels have been found to increase with the use of brain synchronizers, gadgets with flashing lights that are worn like sunglasses during meditation. Raising endorphin levels is bound to make anyone feel better, particularly the genetically addicted, whose endorphin levels are lower than average.

A study on people at risk for AIDS found that a combination of exercise, relaxation therapy, and stress management techniques increased the number of their

T-4 cells, which fight infection and viruses and decrease once the AIDS virus begins to progress. Physical exercise has long been believed to improve a person's resistance to infection, but many recent studies show that extreme forms of exercise are actually an immunosuppressant. Vitamins, on the other hand, enhance the function of the immune system. In one study, supplements of vitamin E and C were given to adults joining an exercise program. Others were given placebos. At the end of six months, there was a significant increase in the number of T lymphocytes in the immune systems of people given the vitamin supplements.

Most interesting to me are the recent findings that have led researchers to postulate that people who are out of touch with their emotions, or unaware of them, or who are unable to express them, particularly the negative ones, are more susceptible to a suppression of the defense capabilities of their immune systems. One study involved volunteers writing down their most traumatic experiences and describing their feelings about them. Many of the subjects had never discussed these experiences of family violence, sexual abuse, suicide attempts, and other upsetting events with anyone. The subjects wrote for four days in succession, for twenty minutes each day, and the study showed a surprising increase in their levels of T-cells. Because food addicts are so good at stuffing down their feelings, they are particularly susceptible to suppression of their immune system's capabilities. Knowing they are actually improving their body's defenses while they are healing emotionally and growing spiritually is one more strong motivation for change.

I am excited about the research that is now being done on the connection between mental state and the immune system, for it takes the whole concept of behavioral medicine out of the realm of superstition and fits it squarely into that of Western medicine. Now, instead of wasting energy on disputing the connection, researchers can concentrate their energies on which behavioral therapies produce the greatest benefit, and on ways to use psychoneuroimmunology in the prevention of disease. Although pharmacologists have yet to produce a synthetic endorphin, we can learn to increase the manufacture of it in our brains by applying the techniques spelled out in this book. They are now all scientifically proven to increase the ability of our immune systems to keep us healthy.

ACTIVITY SIX

Assignment One: Ten Points of Positive Mental Attitude

The following questions will help you to formulate thoughts for an effective life adjustment:

1. Check your personality temperature. Happiness is a byproduct, a result, of effective life adjustment. If you're not happy, what could you do to make your life more fun?
2. Do you have a zest for living? Can you be the developer of excitement and enthusiasm?
3. Are you socially adjusted? Do you like being with and sharing with others?
4. Do you have balance and unity? Balance is needed when you find yourself wrapping your life around one thing or one person. Unity is doing something or not doing something and then refusing to worry about it.
5. Can you live with each problem in your life as it arises? Do you worry about the future or the past? Of all the things you worried about last year, how many of them came true?
6. Do you have insight into your own conduct?

Insight means you know the real underlying reasons for what you do.

7. Do you have a confidential relationship with some other person?
8. Do you have a sense of the ridiculous—of what the world does to you? Can you laugh at yourself? If you look to see who laughs and who doesn't, you need to work in this area of your mental attitude.
9. Are you engaged in satisfying work?
10. Do you know how to worry effectively? Overcome your worries by going to the proper people for help.

Positive self-esteem is the single most important quality in a salesperson, manager, leader, mother, father, or child. It is the feeling that I accept and believe in myself as a changing, imperfect, growing human being. Pride is based on what you have or have done. Self-esteem is based on what you are going to do and what you feel you deserve. I see people holding back because they don't want the loneliness that comes with distancing when you are a winner, but they don't see that farther down toward the finish line there's plenty of company—in the winner's circle.

Remember, you always move toward your dominant thought—every minute of every day. You can't move away from what you're thinking. You move toward your fears just as if they were your goals. You can't dwell on the reverse of an idea. If you're going to motivate your children, your employees, your friends, and yourself, tell yourself what you want and move yourself in the direction of your winning thoughts.

Positive self-motivation is an inner drive, a dissatisfaction with the status quo, a desire for change. It takes place in two prominent emotions: fear in the negative and desire in the affirmative. Fear is the greatest motivator of all, telling you that you have compulsion, which is "have to." Fear is the greatest red light in the world telling you that you can't, which is inhibition. Fear is the strongest compeller and the strongest inhibitor.

Desire is 180 degrees apart from fear and is the greatest propeller. If fear is a compeller, desire is a propeller. Motivation is movement or action toward the current dominant motive.

The winner focuses his intensity on the desired result. You must always focus your intense thought on the reward of success and the place you want to go. You cannot look back, you must look at the focus of the result.

Be willing to dream—to have clearly in mind what it is you want. The mind is the most magnificent biocomputer ever created. It doesn't relate to getting through the day, or being happy, or other general ideas. Winners dream about their goals. They dream specifically with words, pictures, and emotions.

Positive self-direction is focusing on a purpose. If you don't have a purpose, your system will set one for you—to get through the day. It will give you just enough energy to watch TV. The most important thing I've ever found is that if you plan to fail, then fail to plan, and beginning is half done. Beginning anything is half done.

Of all the things I know about living, purpose is the key. People die on purpose, and people die because of no purpose. I heard of a famous personality's saying to his daughter, "I'm tired now, I'm going to do nothing for the rest of my life." He was dead in nine hours. There are two great tragedies in life—never to have had a target and never to have reached it. Reaching your target is up to you.

Goals and dreams need to be internalized. A major key to winning is the internalization of goals, which is known as simulation or self-discipline. Perhaps more than any other characteristic of a winner, the ability to "practice within when you're without" is the key to winning. The imagination is the most powerful tool of all. Winners realize that in your imagination you never have to miss. Every salesperson closes the sale in advance. Every host or hostess plans the party in advance. Winners practice in their imaginations—simulating the winning experience over and over. *Winners in life have persistence. They hang in there.*

A DAY IN THE LIFE

Jenny   *Besides me, there is only one other rebel in the program. His name is Gordon. We talked last night at the coffee machine while everyone else was in Goodnight Group (not for me, thank you very much). Instead of staying alone in my room, I wandered into the alcove where all the goodies are—the decaf coffee, the decaf tea, the packets of bouillon, and the diet sodas and fruit juices we're allowed to snack on. In walks Gordon, and I get all nervous. He's very good looking, and mama, he's got the devil in him. He said he was going to make himself a little espresso and did I want some? Sure, I said. So he rips open four packets of decaf and pours them into the filter of the coffee machine, telling me there is 10 percent caffeine in each pack, so at 40 percent he should get a hit. The espresso was like mud, but it did seem to perk him up. Or maybe it was just a placebo effect. So we got to talking while Goodnight Group was going on. Gordon calls it the Cozy Hour. Every now and then there would be shrieks of laughter from the room, and I mean roars, and I couldn't help but feel like someone on the outside looking in. It's silly for me to feel that way because all I have to do is walk into the group and sit down, but I can't. Oh yes, right, that word's not allowed—I choose not to. For now.*

Six P.M. Well, my new roommate moved in—Martha. She complains about everything and is constantly giving me advice. Why me, Lord? Maybe she's a challenge. I never know what to say to people who bug me.

I just walk away. But you can't use that strategy with a roommate. I'm so frustrated!

•

DAY SEVEN

Step Study: Step Two

"Came to believe that a Power greater than ourselves could restore us to sanity."

When mind and body are at war with each other, they can't work together. Sanity is when the mind, the body, and the spirit are all in harmony, a condition that is not possible as long as a person is in the throes of food addiction.

For years you may have been acknowledging a power greater than your own—your relationship with food. In this program you are asked to consider the possibility of the existence of another power greater than yourself that, unlike the demonic force of your addiction, does not exist to enslave you but to set you free. Step Two is about finding God in other people. It means acknowledging that the power of the group is more powerful than we are, and that we can't do the job of restoring ourselves to sanity alone.

Personality change begins with Step Two, after taking the action of making a life-style change—that is, recognizing we need rituals for contact. In the process of that change, our values, attitudes, and beliefs will be held up to scrutiny, and they will also change. The first to change will be what we value in life. The answer will now be obvious—other people. Those who had valued their isolation because it allowed them to indulge unchecked in their addictive behavior will no longer value it because minus the addiction, isolation is a painful state. There is no joy in it. Suddenly the value of other people, of a supportive group, will increase immeasurably. The attitude of "I can do it myself" will change to "I need other people."

Resisting help from others is resisting help from a higher power, for God works through other people. Faith in a higher power parallels how you trust people in your life. Control means you still don't have trust. As you begin to relinquish that control, you leave room for the power of the group to begin working in you.

Boundaries will also change. Energy will flow in both directions, between you and the fellowship. The power of love is one food addict helping another, and that power will help restore balance in other relationships—between family and friends, and in the workplace. Once the isolation is broken, the new intimacy you will have with the Real You will cause energy to flow in every direction, in every area of your life.

The restoration to sanity is a process. In it, first we come. Our feet bring us, and our unbelieving minds go along for the ride. Then we come to. We wake up. We start feeling. We came, we came to, and we came to believe, hardly an instantaneous event. It takes years for some, much less for others, depending on where they are when their feet first bring them to the process.

Coming to believe in a power greater than ourselves is not necessarily a comforting thought. Any number of horror movies feature powers greater than ourselves. The miracle of the process is that this is a power greater than ourselves that *will restore us to sanity*. What a marvelous thought! The relief of being restored to sanity is greater than any gift a food addict could ask for.

The energy of intimacy, the sharing of the Real Me, is the essence of the Second Step. In the sharing of the Real Me with others, a knowledge of God's energy within your own will protect you. You'll feel empowered, God-protected, nurtured by intimacy. *You won't feel alone.*

The insanity that addictive people feel has a lot to do with the abnormal stress patterns they experience. Normal stress looks like a wavy line—a steady flow of ups and downs. Addictive stress, on the other hand, looks like an erratic heart rate on a cardiologist's screen—constant ups and downs, and finally collapse. At the point of collapse, people look around for a power greater than themselves to restore them to sanity. Some people turn to pills, and the pills usually have side effects. They make them anxious; so they have to take other pills to calm themselves. They in turn make them constipated, listless, dizzy, nauseated, or paranoid; give them tremors, aches, vague feelings of foreboding. The pill takers are always worrying about running out of their prescriptions or not getting a new one filled in time, for they are unable to endure the thought of even a few hours without their pills.

There is only one side effect produced by the restoration of sanity in Step Two, and that is love. We arrive at it through hope and trusting our intuition. What we have been given, we must give back, and we are glad to do so. People are energy through which we can experience love and trust. Think of the infant. Without being able to say a word, it generates incredible energy, and we are fascinated by its purity. We hold it and feel that energy transmitted to us. Similarly, without a word, we encourage others in a state of insanity to seek help, for we bear witness that restoration is possible. We don't need to tell others that we have changed. By the clearness of our eyes and the peacefulness of our spirit, those who knew us when we were troubled will see for themselves that we have been restored to sanity. When we smile at them, we give them hope. We who were so hopeless a short time ago are now joyful, in harmony with ourselves and our surroundings. There is no pill in the universe that can produce this state of mind, only the power that promises to restore us to sanity.

Food addicts arrive at Step Two feeling disillusioned,

angry, and betrayed. Have they gone through the pain and humiliation of admitting their powerlessness over food to be hit on the head with the need to believe in God? These days, it's easy to feel morally superior to the whole idea of religion. The ghastly religious wars of the Middle East make many people want to reject the idea of God altogether. In fact, the entire history of religion with its trail of blood and tears thousands of years in duration is enough to turn people away entirely.

No wonder so many people have problems with God. Fortunately, God doesn't have problems with them. The God of the 12-step program has no ulterior motive, no hidden agenda, no temple that needs financing, no ring that needs to be kissed. You who have problems with God can decide the word stands for "good orderly direction," or that the power greater than yourselves is the power of the support group, or the power of this book if it's helping you feel better about yourself. The problems most people have with the idea of power is they have been taught to fear it, for it always implies power over—where the strong take advantage of the weak. The power of the 12-step program is never about power over. It's never something that needs to be feared. It empowers. It brings people from the state of powerlessness to being given power through others, by sharing the intimacy of who you really are. It's about becoming "happy, joyous, and free." It's about achieving a positive state of mind in which, wherever you are, whomever you're with, whatever you're doing, you will feel good about yourself because you know and love who you are, and because you will feel the presence of God in your life.

Sane people don't go on crusades. They just go about the business of living. Sane people don't have a yen to control your mind. They've learned they don't want to control anything, not even their own minds. They've learned to give up the entire idea of control and to wait in that naked and vulnerable state for a power greater than themselves that will give them something much better than they could ever have created on their own, something they most likely have never even experienced, or felt only in small moments of bliss.

The precious gift of awareness is waiting for those who come to believe. There is no price to pay, no pledge of allegiance, no vows, no dues or initiation fees, no contracts to sign. All that is required is belief, and somehow that comes. Sometimes it seems to come of its own accord. The power we seek does not always manifest itself in a shaft of light, although that happens. I have heard too many sane, normal, ordinary people tell about that experience to doubt it. The power manifests itself when we pray not for what we want but merely for the power to carry out God's will for us, having the faith of a mustard seed.

Belief is a matter of "reliance, not defiance." It does not tell God what to do and then get angry when it doesn't happen. That you have to give up your list of demands—what your own will thinks you want—may seem the most bitter pill of all to swallow, but I can assure you God's will for you is like a surprise gift containing something you didn't even know you wanted, but badly needed and never thought to ask for, and never dreamed could be yours. The room for surprise once you step out of God's way is one of the most intriguing aspects of this program. The power that comes when you ask for knowledge of God's will is another. Following it is so easy, like having the wind at your back instead of fighting it every inch of the way. There is little more I can say until you experience for yourself that there is a healing power greater than your own, except my constant reassurance that help is on the way, if you will just keep going in the direction you're in. The disease of addiction is a detour from the person we were meant to be. Recovery is a discovery process of who that wonderful person really is through a personal revelation of God's will for you.

The experience of slogging on without reason to believe is called faith, and it is a state of grace. In that protective state, faith will carry you until you find your first tangible evidence that this program works. How will you know when it starts working? You will *feel* it, and that feeling will be all the proof you will need to continue.

═══════════

ACTIVITIES FOR DAY SEVEN

Assignment One: My Concept of a Higher Power

Draw a picture of the God of your childhood. Describe your relationship with that God. Draw a picture of a higher power that you would like to believe in. Do you believe there is or might be a power greater than yourself? If not, do you wish you could believe there was a power greater than yourself? If you are still filled with doubt and despair, are you willing to continue reading this book in spite of your objections to the "God stuff"? Be honest. The only one this answer is important to is you. God will wait.

Assignment Two: Prayer Is When You Listen

The terrible emptiness addicts feel that they are compelled to fill with something outside themselves—a substance, activity, relationships—is the absence of their energy, spirit. Once they abstain from their obsession, that void can feel intolerable for a while. No matter where they go, they feel no one's there. Nothing they do or say is of any significance.

"A cup must be empty to be filled." Once it is drained of all illusions and false securities, it can be replenished, with your real spirit. The more expressive you become, the more spiritual you are. The essence of spirituality at Janet Greeson's "Your Life Matters" is that we help people empty themselves so there is room for their spirit, their real energy, to fill the void. This is in no way a religious program. It's more about expression of energy. Birds sing, dogs bark. We are multifaceted expressions of energy. Religion is about dogma and ritual. Spirituality is about becoming positive, creative, loving, and enthusiastic human beings. The Greek derivation of the word "enthusiasm" is "God in me." That's the energy within you waiting to be tapped, waiting to be released.

I like to think of the word "God" as meaning "good orderly direction." The direction is not to follow a leader but the still, small voice that speaks to us when we listen, the light we see, the energy we express, the one we know without knowing is our higher self. Addiction is a detour away from that person, and recovery is a rediscovery of who we would have been, had our addiction not gotten in the way.

The Twelve Steps and Twelve Traditions of Alcoholics Anonymous say, "In every case, pain has been the price of admission into the new life." The intolerable pain of addiction compels people to seek a way other than their own, for it becomes obvious to them that their way is not working. Surrender of self-will is all that needs to be done to get in touch with a power higher than ourselves. That power will not come knocking on your door, but those who acknowledge their powerlessness are amazed at how readily it responds.

Surrender is not giving up but giving in—to make room for a powerful source of love and nurturance that will help you if you only ask. The miracle of this program is that we can change. We were not put on this earth to suffer but to be "happy, joyous, and free." A 12-step program is a blueprint for that. It has no leaders or holy gurus, no hierarchy, no promotional gimmicks. No one ever got rich or famous exploiting it. It does not even advertise that it exists, but people in pain find it and get better. You can, too.

The following is a prayer commonly used at 12-step meetings. Because it is so familiar, the meaning behind the words has lost its impact. I have supplied you with a meditation on what the words might mean to you in order to restore the power of its message. Repeat the prayer and meditation out loud before you go to bed so its message can penetrate your conscious defenses as you fall asleep.

THE LORD'S PRAYER

Our Father . . .
A genderless word, the source of unconditional love we may never have had from another human being, a parent to the needy child within us.

Which art in heaven . . .
Not a place in the sky or an afterlife, but now, within us, waiting to be occupied.

Hallowed be thy name . . .
As soon as the power of this source of universal love is made abstract by giving it a name, it can be abused by those who would claim it, proselytize, and brutalize others who call it by a different name.

Thy kingdom come . . .
To heal this suffering world we live in.

Thy will be done on earth as it is in heaven . . .
My will has enslaved me. Your will is to set me free.

Give us this day our daily bread . . .
Enough for today, no need for a surplus that can be hoarded, bought, and sold. One day at a time you give me all I need if I only ask, and tomorrow you will give again.

And forgive us our trespasses . . .

You don't speak of sins but of boundaries I have crossed.

As we forgive those who trespass against us . . .

Having been so readily forgiven by you for violating the boundaries of others, I return the favor. I hold no ill will in order to leave room for love.

And lead us not into temptation . . .

I am tested every day. You will lead me down another, safer path if I ask you every day.

But deliver us from evil . . .

You are there to protect me from the destructiveness of negativity, both within me and all around me. You will keep me safe if I ask you every day.

For thine is the kingdom . . .

Not mine, or anyone else's who seeks to own it, for it is not a place to be owned.

The power . . .

For You do not abuse it.

And the glory . . .

For which I freely give credit where it's due, to save myself from the enslavement of grandiosity.

Forever and ever . . .

The world will not come to an end. It will go through changes but it will not die.

Amen.

Assignment Three: The Sixty Percent

Ten percent of the way people experience you is about your body, your physical self; 30 percent of it is your mind, the way you think, feel, and express yourself; and the remaining 60 percent is your spirit. What is the spirit? It is something only you can feel or be aware of because it is inside of you. It goes by many names: your positive energy, your essence, your godliness, your inner child, your being, your life force.

Addicts become disconnected from their spirit and turn to something outside of themselves. But the cost of this false energy is high, and it ultimately fails us. I have seen certain people come into treatment so dispirited they have no energy at all. Our job is to get them reconnected to their spirit.

You can uncover this ball of fire, this wondrous "beingness" that is buried within you. This is what recovery is all about. Once I became reconnected with my spirit, I was very comfortable wherever I went. For me it was finding a place for myself in this world, knowing I'm not better than anyone else, nor am I any worse. I'm just as good as the next guy. Once I reconnected with my spirit, every day was full of joy. I was no longer a prisoner to my addiction; I was free to live.

One of the most effective ways to coax this spirit of yours to come forth is through dance. Because it is a nonverbal form of expression, it circumvents the intellect and all its critical inhibitors. The impulse to dance comes straight from the spirit, for it yearns to express itself. Here is one way to make your spirit feel safe enough to express itself: dance alone in the privacy of your bedroom wearing earphones, or turn the music up good and loud. Now close your eyes to prevent that critical mind from observing your dancing. Listen to the music and let it move you. Let it really move you—your hands, your arms, your feet, knees, legs, hips, head, and shoulders. Keep dancing wildly until you feel the exultation of your spirit. Let it go free. It's been confined for so long!

A DAY IN THE LIFE

Martha   Well, I feel a little better today, Dear Diary. The throbbing headache is finally gone. My eyesight seems to have improved, although I know that can't be so. Let's say I see a little clearer, without so much fogginess. Funny how I didn't even know the fog was there until it lifted.

Just seven days away from my life and I can look at it a little more objectively. It looks pretty grim to me. How could I have let myself fall apart like this? It's not like I haven't been working on my issues for years. I started my incest survivor's group, and I've had three different therapists. Why can't I change? What's stopping me? I'm scared, but scared of what? That feeling of being scared looms over me at all times. It makes me kind of cower when I walk. I'm always watching out of the corner of my eye. I'm always ready to bolt out the door or up the stairs. The thing is, I've talked about my mother's abuse and my uncle's abuse for years, but it all remained in my head. The words were just words that came out of my mouth; the feelings all stayed inside. Here, it's when I watch and listen to others talk about their experiences that I feel the deepest for myself. I have to hear the words and the feelings of the other patients in order to feel them for myself. It's a beginning, I guess.

But I feel so lonely here. I try to be helpful and friendly, but people ignore me. When Chuck walks into the dining room, everybody says, "Hey Chuck, there's a place over here." When I walk toward a table with my tray, nobody says anything. I don't understand. I have never understood. Maybe I'm just a basically unappealing person. Maybe it's the way I look. Oh, I can't stand feeling this way anymore. I've got to change.

Please God, help me, I'm so scared and terrified!

•

5

Week Two: Communicating

The first days of treatment are a disorienting time, due to the combined effects of substance withdrawal and the exposure to new ideas and a loving, caring, nonjudgmental environment. By the end of the third day, patients may come out of the throbbing fog of withdrawal, take a look around at the real world, and shut down in fear and denial. We want to keep the energy flow open so that they can experience being in a safe place. If we penetrate their defenses, patients often say they start to feel better.

Chuck, Jenny, and Martha are each typical in their own way. Chuck's defenses are the most successful because they still work for him. People seek him out. Chuck is a natural first-born leader. But Chuck is reaching the point where he is getting desperate about his need to change. He has seen his need to be good from a new perspective; he knows it is a defense mechanism. He has also learned in his group that feelings can emerge and be discussed and and that it is safe for him to do so. He has learned, to his surprise, that those feelings don't hurt as much after being discussed.

Martha is having a particularly difficult time. Her resistance is great, and unlike Chuck's defensive good guy image, Martha's form of defense doesn't win her any popularity contests. Martha is a control freak. She has to keep the lid on tight, or she will blow, and that lid is starting to jiggle. She radiates anger, and her sense of self is distorted. While the other patients see her as a pain, Martha sees herself as the knowing one. She consistently tries to help others and puts their needs before her own, but only to fulfill her need to control. When she isn't actively trying to help others, she is giving unasked-for advice. Unfortunately, the help she gives is what *she* decides is needed.

Nevertheless, something is stirring in Martha also. She has abruptly left the room on several occasions when the issue of childhood sexual abuse came up, because she has a great fear of releasing her tears. But the nurses have reported she cries out in her sleep, and twice she has been found weeping alone. Although Martha has always known about her uncle's sexual abuse (unlike some survivors, she did not bury the repeated incidents), she minimized it for years and then in her incest survivor's group could not express any feelings other than anger.

The staff's goal this week for Martha's treatment—and for Chuck's, Jenny's, and all the patients'—is to promote a feeling of safety by providing a loving, caring, and supportive environment. Special emphasis will be placed on assisting Martha to experience how others perceive her. Unlike Gordon, who is charming even when outrageous, Martha's defenses only serve to isolate her further, as patients withdraw from her unpleasantness.

Another goal to pursue with Martha is to help her see that her defensive need for control is keeping her stuck. As her secrets are being shaken by people openly talking about themselves as victims of incest, Martha's need for control has become desperate in the extreme.

The roots of Jenny's depression are more difficult to

probe at this point in treatment. The incident on the first day with the roommate who made a racial comment—even though Jenny brushed it aside and was appreciative of the response of staff and patients—must have shaken her trust on a deep level. It was a particularly vulnerable moment to have been confronted with that kind of cruelty.

Jenny identifies with the Lost Child, the person in the family who is ignored, and whose depression has no known cause, unlike the victims of childhood abuse. The situation that propelled her into treatment—a failed love affair, the death of a dog, a bad experience at a weekend retreat—do not seem "enough" to her, compared to the awful stories she has been hearing from other patients. She just wants to fade away.

Jenny is more well liked than she realizes, but she holds herself at a distance from the others. She has developed close relationships only with people in her group and with her primary therapist. She has a way of slipping out of meetings when people show strong feelings and has expressed her feelings only on one occasion, in a psychodrama session when she heard a patient tell of being abandoned at the age of four. As the person described sitting patiently on a park bench at the zoo for hours with her baby brother and waiting for her mother to come back, Jenny became tearful. At the encouragement of the others, she began to sob deeply. When her emotions had subsided, she said she felt very tired and went to her room. In the following days she began to withdraw from everyone except Gordon, with whom she has formed a kind of "outsider" alliance.

During this second week the focus will be on improving communications. Having experienced themselves without their defenses, the patients are highly motivated to continue exploring alternatives, especially expressing their feelings in new ways that can be experienced by others rather than taking the usual reactive defense. Allowing our newly emerging real selves the opportunity to develop new communication skills is an important tool in the recovery process.

NOURISHING THE BODY

If major depression is eating you, treatment at "Your Life Matters" accelerates recovery. At home, change will come about more slowly. Nevertheless, during your first week certain changes may already be evident: After seven days of following the food plan and abstaining from refined sugar, white flour, and caffeine, you must also be feeling quite differently about yourself. You may be noticing a diminishing of your obsession with food, particularly binge items, and a return of your morning appetite. Caffeine withdrawal rarely lasts more than a week, so you may already be enjoying the serenity and clearheadedness that comes after that drug has been flushed from your system.

You may also be noticing an improvement in your general mood. The empty feeling caused by bingeing, sugar, and caffeine may no longer be with you much of the time. Its lifting may be so gradual, and your acceptance of depression as your normal state so complete, that you may not even notice its absence for a while. You may be particularly aware of your new state of mind when you first wake up in the morning and in the late afternoon, when you were used to boosting your sagging mood with a jolt of caffeine and sugar. Your body is already thanking you even if your mind hasn't caught on to what you're doing yet.

In early abstinence, people often feel annoyed in the presence of those who do obsess about food. They, on the other hand, are not going to be happy about the decision you have made because it magnifies their problem. This is a difficult period, and the stress of being around people who are still bingeing may be too great. I suggest you avoid your eating buddies for a short time.

YOU ARE A CELEBRATION OF LIFE

After saying your affirmations regularly for seven days, you will also be experiencing the first effects of positive self-talk. When you wake up in the morning, instead of the usual dread, you may be feeling a peaceful anticipation of the day. This is your subconscious mind at work, already processing the new messages it is so hungry to receive. Every now and then you may experience something someone once called a "s'mor," a "small moment of rapture." This feeling, brief though it may be, is a preview of the state of mind that is rightfully yours to own, the kind of feeling that should be constant merely for experiencing the miracle of being alive. When you feel a s'mor, know your positive self-talk is beginning to work and that, with continued practice, many more good feelings will follow. If you've rarely felt good about yourself, be prepared for the shock of it, and when it comes, don't reject it—rub it in! It's your birthright, no matter what kind of destructive messages you gave yourself in the past.

MEDITATION IS WHEN YOU LISTEN

In the beginning, meditating is an act of will—willing the mind to settle, the body to quiet, controlling thoughts as they pass in and out of consciousness. With patient practice, that need to control disappears, and the meditation process begins to work. Put your concentration on your breathing when the board meeting in your head is convened. Don't try to discourage all the cross-conversation, just blow it away with your breath. Orient yourself to your surroundings. Think of your feet as being conduits of energy from the ground that flows through your body and leaves through the top of your head. You are a receptor, listening for, not sending, messages. When those messages begin to be heard, they may be wordless. Sometimes they will take a visual form. Other times they will just be a feeling of quietude. You may not be aware of the answer when it fills your mind, only when you act on it. Suddenly you stop and say to yourself, "Why didn't I think of that before? How simple!"

In the beginning, you may be able to tolerate only a few minutes of meditation at a time. Don't worry about duration for now, just keep to a daily schedule and the time will extend itself.

YOU'VE GOT TO MOVE YOUR BODY

One week of regular exercise is too brief a time for much to be happening to your body aside from some sore muscles, but you may assume that part of your new tranquillity is the result of the twenty to thirty minutes a day you are exercising. You may want to think about incorporating a new form of exercise into your daily routine, now that you have found how simple and pleasurable it is to make room for it, but remember, wherever you are and however busy you get, a half hour of brisk walking is always possible.

HUGS

If you're not making an effort to reach out to others, the changes you are making will be superficial and won't last. Because addiction is a disease of isolation, once you give up your love affair with a substance, your emptiness will drive you to despair unless you replace your loss with meaningful contact with the outside world. After a week of attending Anonymous meetings, you may already be feeling the urge to go up to newcomers and make them feel welcome. That urge is the healing message of this program already at work. The good that comes to you from it must be passed on in order for it to grow.

Other addicts readily understand the anguish of being alone while surrounded by people. Making the first move, establishing eye contact, and giving a hug sound so simple to accomplish, but to beginners still imprisoned in their isolation like you may have been just last week, breaking out is a seemingly impossible act of will. You know you're on the road to recovery when you first reach out to help someone else. If hugs don't come easy to you yet, or if you feel they are not always appropriate, try embracing with your eyes or a smile or the words "How are things going for you?" In the process, you will be infused with healing energy, an octane that will fill the uncomfortable void caused by the acknowledgment of your powerlessness. That power from without will fuel your recovery. You can't possibly experience it until you have shared or connected yourself to others. As long as we remain self-obsessed, the obsession blocks our energy and makes it difficult to relate to others. All our lives we have been blaming our bodies for our not getting the right mate, the promotion, or success on the playing field of life. As long as we scapegoated our bodies, we could avoid taking responsibility for our communication styles and personalities. No addict wants to take responsibility, but it must be done.

"Experience and express" is the theme of the second week of treatment as we proceed on the path to intimacy. Acknowledging and moving through the pain of emptiness is essential to recovery. When you begin to tell yourself the pain is unendurable, think of it as childbirth. You are in a similar process, giving birth to your true nature, and there is no change without pain. I assure you it will pass.

DAY EIGHT

Changing

It might seem to you as though you have to change everything. The most difficult part is *making the decision* to change. Putting off making a decision is making a decision not to make a decision. I know it's hard to change, and yet it is the very thing required of us. Assisting us are many tools and techniques, one of them being self-examination. The assignment for today is an extended evaluation, not only of your own life changes so far, but those of the members of your immediate family. Only within this larger context can hidden patterns of behavior be detected and "blind spots" camouflaged by denial be seen, so that the bigger picture can be complete and meaningful.

ACTIVITIES FOR DAY EIGHT

Assignment One: "The Life Changes Scale"

The following is a helpful assessment tool called "The Life Changes Scale."* Completing and charting this

* "The Life Changes Scale" was written by Tom M. Saunders, Ph.D. Dr. Saunders is a counseling psychologist in private practice in Winter Park, Florida. He is president and founder of The Chrysalis Foundation, Inc., which provides training in family systems throughout the country. This excerpt is reprinted by permission.

scale will help you to better understand the underpinnings of your present communication patterns and how they have developed.

———— THE LIFE CHANGES SCALE ————

Please make one copy of this scale for each member of your family age ten or older to complete. Each question means exactly what each family member perceives it to mean.

Write three answers in the space provided for each question.

In the blank to the left of each answer, write the number of the year that you would most associate with each answer.

When you have completed each answer with an associated year, follow the instructions at the end for charting your answers.

Name your three most intimate friends.

_____ 1) _____

_____ 2) _____

_____ 3) _____

Name your three most passionate enemies.

_____ 4) _____

_____ 5) _____

_____ 6) _____

Name your three most memorable incidents.

——— 7) _____

——— 8) _____

——— 9) _____

Name your three illnesses of choice (what are your "target organs"? to what does your body usually succumb?).

——— 10) _____

——— 11) _____

——— 12) _____

Name your three most important personal issues under the category of "unfinished business."

——— 13) _____

——— 14) _____

——— 15) _____

Name your three greatest losses.

——— 16) _____

——— 17) _____

——— 18) _____

Name your three most significant geographical moves.

——— 19) _____

——— 20) _____

——— 21) _____

Name your three greatest fears.

_____ 22) _____

_____ 23) _____

_____ 24) _____

Name your three favorite forms of dependency.

_____ 25) _____

_____ 26) _____

_____ 27) _____

Name your three best defenses (major life excuses used most often to avoid responsibility).

_____ 28) _____

_____ 29) _____

_____ 30) _____

INSTRUCTIONS FOR CHARTING:

Draw a scale using the model as an example.

On the left end of the scale, print "BIRTH" and write your Month, Day, and Year of Birth.

On the right end of the scale, print "PRESENT" and write today's Month, Day, and Year.

Take each item # from the questionnaire, and place it on the scale. Use the Year which you assigned to each item # as a way of locating its relative position on the scale.

See the example below!

Month & Day of Birth				Today's Month & Day

	#2	#1	#3	#4	
BIRTH					**PRESENT**
Year of Birth	1	1	1	1	Today's Year
	9	9	9	9	
	4	5	6	8	
	7	6	4	4	

© The Chrysalis Foundation, Inc., 1987

Name your three most intimate friends.

<u>1956</u> 1) Rhonda

<u>1947</u> 2) Christine

<u>1964</u> 3) Gerry

Name your three most passionate enemies.

<u>1984</u> 4) Marge

Assignment Two: Interpreting "The Life Changes Scale"

How You Respond

As you have recently learned, one of *your* rights is to be responsible for how you perceive and report an experience. There are no hidden meanings in "The Life

Changes Scale." The results are today's snapshot of how you view your life to date and what it means to you now. If you would like to discover where your important changes fit with those of your family members, you may wish to copy this scale and give it to the important members of your family network to complete, then compare results with them at a later time.

As you recall, the instructions reminded you, "Each question means exactly what each family member perceives it to mean." Some of the descriptors may seem a little strange at first. Perhaps you have never considered "passionate" as an adjective for "enemies." But passionate is a good synonym for "intense," and generally, when we are busy assigning those feelings that we do not wish to own as the property of another, we become passionately involved in that process of blaming.

"Illnesses of *choice*" is another uncommon phrase. Few would acknowledge ever electing illness, yet none would deny that the daily stress, fatigue, and improper nourishment with which we punish our physical body must undermine the immune system, and handicap it at best.

The "Year" assigned in the blank to the left of each numbered item is a "best guess" as to the year that we associate with that item becoming important in our lives. Again, being exact is not important.

As always, your conscious judgmental mind has done its best to interfere with your response to each item. For those persons who have learned to be afraid of being responsible for their "Rights," the words of the cartoon character Pogo could not be more correct: "We have met the enemy, and they is us!" For this reason, you may want to wait a few days, and then complete "The Life Changes Scale" a second time; the results will be quite different if you follow your heart, and respond in writing to the first flash of a response that comes to your mind.

Charting the Results

Draw a scale like the one in the example, but allow yourself more room. On the left end of the scale is the date of *your birth,* perhaps the most important day of your life! At the right end of the scale is today's date, the second most important day of your life.

Commencing with item #1 and the Year assigned to that item, estimate approximately where that year would fall on the scale between your birth year and now. Write the year just below the scale, as shown in the example, and the corresponding item number just above the scale. Continue, in the same manner, with each item until all thirty items have been charted.

Discovering the Clusters

As you review the results of your charting, you will notice that *changes* usually do not happen in "ones." Changes will usually occur in groups.

Circle any Year or Years that have two or more items assigned to them. As you remember that year, at this moment, try to recall any other significant changes that happened during that same approximate time span.

For those of you who have asked other family members to complete this exercise, when they have finished all of the above, compare notes with them. Do any of your significant years of change correspond with theirs? It will be helpful to hear their perceptions of what was happening during those important years as well. In this way, you will begin to better understand the significant events in your life as well as the backdrop against which they happened.

Just as in the solar system or the atom, each particle is in delicate balance with every other particle. No one family member ever goes through a transition that does not in some way affect every other family member in the system.

What Does It All Mean?

"The Life Changes Scale" was first developed in 1987 as a research tool for The Chrysalis Foundation, Inc., of Winter Park, Florida. Chrysalis's President/Founder, Tom M. Saunders, Ph.D., has worked with families for over twenty years, and currently maintains a private practice in Florida called Family Systems Consultants.

Through the years, Dr. Saunders had observed that when family members were seen individually and made excellent progress over a period of time, their progress was often limited by the onset of other problems in the family. A teenager who had been acting out, now back on a positive track, was followed into treatment by a depressed mother. By the time the mother had harnessed her creativity and was actively pursuing a more fulfilling life, her husband would have a heart attack, thereby forcing the oldest child to return home from college to help support the family.

At first, these "coincidences" were discarded as projections of the therapist, and ignored. However, when the same patterns were observed over a period of years in one family after another, interested colleagues began to join Dr. Saunders in the research effort.

Of all their findings the most fascinating is perhaps the "ethernet phenomenon." Remember the bump-um cars at the county fair? Those cars were powered by electricity through a pole at the rear of the car that reached to touch an electrical net about eight feet overhead. When one car would strike another hard enough to jar it off the net, the car would not be operational until it was pushed back into place, touching the net once again.

Familes appear to be connected by such an energy net—a sixth sense, an unconscious, spiritual electrical field through which all important communication takes place. Through work with both Chrysalis and Family

Systems Consultants, Dr. Saunders has discovered that family members, though separated by geographical boundaries, emotional isolation, and lack of physical communication, still experience their major clusters of changes during the same periods of time, plus or minus six months. Even those family members who have not spoken for periods of twenty years or more will encounter the same changes, just as if there had been an ongoing dialogue.

It is interesting to note that most people do not believe in this familial connection when they first hear about it. Yet those same individuals are quick to acknowledge that all animals and probably most children have such sixth-sense information available. Few, regardless of their scientific persuasions, would try to fool a Doberman or horse of whom they were afraid.

The Meaning of Change

Change is healthy. Change is necessary. Change must involve dying and being reborn. Change, by definition, means taking a new risk and being responsible for the consequences.

However, as alluded to earlier, individual change never happens in a vacuum. When one member of a family risks doing anything substantially different, the entire family system must begin to adjust, ever so slightly, to accommodate that new change.

The most natural reaction of any family system, however, is to try to maintain the "status quo" at any cost! The family will almost always try, at an unconscious level, to pull the changing member back into his or her old behavior, even though the support of the family is critical if that change is to remain for any length of time.

A parallel phenomenon exists in the overnight religious conversion. Swept up in a powerful emotional tidal wave, these individuals, surrounded by enormous love and support, make a decision to change their way of living in favor of gaining more of this support from others. However, when they return home, their family and friends still see them as they were and treat them as they always have. Any positive change, because of the powerful pull of the family, becomes difficult to maintain.

Enslavement or Isolation

Part of the value of identifying these personal and family changes is that it allows us to better understand the impact that these changes have had upon the individual, and the system of which he or she is a part. Losing weight, as an example, has far greater impact than those shed pounds. It means giving up an entire role, a place in the sun, if you will—a direct link to a special relationship to at least one member of the family, and usually several others.

Liz's story is a good example. Her mother has been tracking her weight since Liz was in junior high. With the same zeal as the spouse of an alcoholic who counts drinks and bottles, Mom has always been chiding Liz about how much she eats, how little she eats, how many diets she has tried, and so on. Yet, any substantial loss of weight has always been put down with sarcasm.

Liz's father doesn't say much. He began to touch Liz inappropriately just about the same time that Liz began to obsess about weight. Liz has avoided her father ever since and has never told Mom because it could mean that her parent's underground cold war could become a divorce. To make matters worse, Liz's brother, five years her senior, came home quite drunk one evening, accidentally got into bed with Liz, and blacked out.

Liz has "swallowed" everything and kept the family secrets intact. However, the sad implication of her losing her weight is that she fears losing both her parents, their marriage, and her older brother at the same time. While not all family dynamics are as tragic, the implication of enslavement or isolation is a part of every family. If we do whatever seems necessary to save our family and keep them intact, we become enmeshed with them to a point of losing our own identity. At the other extreme, if we attempt to take care of our own needs, we risk isolation.

Who we are, and how we are, is always a part of this ongoing paradox. Our level of assertive communication relates directly, at any given moment, to where we are in this process of separating ourselves from our original family system. Ironically, wherever we happen to become stuck in this process is the role that we continue to play and replay in every social system of which we become a part, including marriage.

A Change of Role, a Change in Communication

What must become obvious by now is that how we communicate is a direct representation of the role that we have elected to play in our family, our work life, our social setting, and our marriage. Don't ever be fooled by passive persons telling you that they have no power, but truly wish for some. When passive persons can't decide where they would like to eat, someone will either rise to the occasion to make the decision for them, feed them, or leave them to their own devices to starve to death. Most passive people get fed. That's power!

If you have trouble believing in the "ethernet" concept—that what looks like coincidence is actually an unconscious energy connection between closely bonded people that results in a reaction to every action—think about how all of the matched pairs in the world find each other.

For the aggressive person who likes to bulldoze and run other people's lives, there are always others available who just can't wait to be told what to do, all the while complaining bitterly about their lot in life. However, the best part of having your life run for you is that there is only a minimal level of responsibility to meet, such as hygiene, tying your shoes, and the like.

The passive–aggressive person obviously needs to be matched with someone adequately skilled in the same intricate dance. These individuals are usually more exciting since they play many roles, of either variety, and can turn on a dime, if necessary, to change directions. The bad news is that when you have seen their performance, it's time to move on to another relationship.

To be assertive is to risk change. Like most quality spices, a little goes a long way. One of the early faults of assertiveness training was that the newly skilled pledges would leave their classrooms, rear their heads, and assert all over anyone around them in the name of changing their role. For the unsuspecting spouse or friends, this often meant the death of a relationship because the newly assertive person had never bothered to understand the power of the unresolved anger cooking just below the surface.

Permanent Change Is Gradual

If you have ever tried to change a golf or tennis swing, you know it takes a great deal of practice to program the brain. Changing roles means risking a new role time and time again until it begins to become familiar.

It was the French philosopher and scientist Pascal who wrote one of the most interesting things I've read about change. Pascal said that not believing in God had no consequences if there were no God. But if there were a God, he continued to reason, then everything would be in favor of being a believer.

Hedging his bet, Pascal said that at the point of confessing to believe in God, the new believer must act *as if* there is a God. One must pray *as if* prayer will be answered, kneel *as if* one is humble, and in doing so, obtain faith.

Permanent change is accomplished in just such tiny steps. Each day, each hour, each moment, must be lived *as if* the responsible change is possible, *and in that moment, change occurs!*

A DAY IN THE LIFE

Chuck *This assignment is really getting me upset. I'm supposed to be the one with needs for a twenty-four-hour period and everybody around here is cooperating a bit much, focusing on me and my needs! If I so much as ask, "How are you today?" I get this look and a response of "How are you?" I tell you, what is really starting to emerge, though, while I stew in this new role, is a new dark side beyond my addiction, beyond my parents, to the way I experience the world. I know now that what I need more than anything (because I already have love) is acceptance. I need to be seen by the world for who I am and not what I look like. I told that need to Jenny and she understood. We cried together. In the eyes of the world I'm a fat man and she's a woman of color. But we're not adjectives. One word can't describe us. We're much more complicated than that.*

I'm getting close to individual people here like Jenny and others, especially my roommate Gordon, who's so unstable and out of control most of the time, it's hard to catch on to who he really is. But I know who he really is, just like I know who Jenny really is. In group I have seen Gordon turn into a toddling little boy bawling so hard it touched my heart, and when the therapist asked him afterwards to choose one of us to comfort him, he came to me, and now he's my kid brother.

Funny thing though, when he asked me this afternoon about what I needed from him, I snapped. Too much changing for me to take in. I've got to bring up in group what I felt when Gordon became my kid brother. We've got to talk about the three kids and sick brother and five grandkids and four cats and two dogs and a very needy neighbor. I don't want to be Chuck the great guy any more because the load is too heavy, and yet it's the role that gives me the most satisfaction in life. Do I have to deny myself that, too?

•

=========

DAY NINE

Defense Mechanisms

Our minds may deceive us, but our bodies never lie. The autonomic nervous system has a life of its own and pays no attention to what the mind wants to project to the outside world. When it feels like blushing, it blushes. When it feels like crying, it cries. When it's alarmed, it breaks out in gooseflesh. Because of this truth-telling disparity between mind and body, when people come into treatment, we watch as much as we listen. Their actions speak so loudly we can hardly hear a word they're saying, and we know that no matter what they try to convey to us with words, their nonverbal language tells the truth.

Some are full of shame. Their eyes are cast down, they readily weep, they cover their face with their hands when they talk as if they had something to hide, they are angry at themselves and feel empty or numb. The very obese are often suicidally depressed. Nothing seems to work for them now, and they have completely submerged their identity under layers of fat. The heaviest patient I ever had weighed 470 pounds. She was barely able to get herself dressed and thought she had no reason for living except to eat herself to death.

Most people come in depressed. Some are hostile, blaming others for their problems, angry at everyone but themselves and full of complaints. Gerald G. Jampolsky, M.D., author of *Teach Only Love,* remarks, "The most offensive patients are the ones who need the most love." Sometimes that's difficult to remember, but I've never failed to acknowledge the truth of that statement.

Still other people are placid. They will calmly tell you there's nothing the matter with them except a need to control their weight. They will go out of their way to please people and do whatever they can to get approval.

Surprisingly, the passive people are the most difficult to treat, for there is no struggle. The shame-based people are struggling with themselves, the anger-based people are struggling against the world, but the passive people-pleasers are not struggling against anything. They want somebody to fix them without taking action themselves.

In order to get the passive types to work, we have to shake them up a bit. We don't respond to their need to please. Getting them to drop their defensive behavior is no game; if we can't shake them out of their passivity, they usually go home without doing any real work on their emotions and don't get better. What I do is make them into bad patients. I'm always glad when I see their anger and feistiness begin to come out. My nurses say they don't like them as well as they did when they first came on the unit, but that's okay by me. They're learning to challenge and create boundaries, developing an identity beyond just being nice.

People who are full of guilt and shame often don't know why, or give erroneous reasons for the way they feel. In their intake interview they may deny or claim they are not aware of anything in their childhood that caused them to feel so bad about themselves, but the red flag is up to look for abuse. These people are often the ones who go right to work. As soon as they begin to respond to a safe and loving environment, they are so needy and grateful they begin to express their pain.

Passive people, on the other hand, are so numb their deep-seated pain needs time to surface, and much is done during treatment to stimulate it to rise. In the words of the psychotherapist Dr. Elvin Semrod, "When you feel nothing, *that's* when you hurt the most."

Before angry people can get down to work, they must struggle through their denial. They may refuse to admit that they are the problem or even that they have one, but once they do, the energy is there to work with. When I was counseling in Navy alcohol treatment centers, I found the people who were referred against their will actually did better than the ones who came into treatment voluntarily. The recalcitrant ones were constantly telling me, "Screw you, I'm no alkie," while the people who came into treatment on their own weren't struggling with their denial at all.

There is often a secondary denial that lies beneath the surface of an open admission of addiction. Sometimes this denial emerges when a person returns home after treatment, when it might lead to a relapse. I often wonder if people openly in denial get a lot more attention by therapists during treatment and consequently may avoid having to go through the anguish of secondary denial.

Kinds of Defenses

The behaviors people use as defense mechanisms keep the world at arm's length and their true feelings buried. *Blaming* is a form of protection. People who play the victim role are often rigid in their belief that the world is out to get them, and they are never the reason for their problems. I like to tell people that every time I point a finger at you, there are three fingers pointing back at me. I recognize a fault in you because I have it in me, and that makes me mad! *Judging* is a related form of defense. Those who are the harshest judges of others are also the hardest on themselves, and this provides a clue to work with them on elevating their self-esteem.

Patronizing is a favorite defense of those who feel inferior to others. They project a false sense of superiority for protection. Patronizing is especially common among patients who hold some status in the outside world. They wear their arrogance as a mask until they feel safe enough to discard it. Others use *intellectualizing, explaining,* and *justifying,* doing a lot of verbal gymnastics to avoid identifying their feelings. They are often skilled at another defense, *generalizing.*

Projecting is another common defense mechanism. People who use it will confront others for something they do themselves. Whenever a patient becomes upset over the behavior of another patient in treatment, it usually means they are observing what they don't like about themselves.

Smiling and *complying* are defenses used a lot by people-pleasers. *Withdrawing* or going into a deep *depression* are defenses used by passive types, who work hard at making people guess what's wrong with them. They may get annoyed when I tell them, "I'm not a good guesser. You'll have to *tell* me what's wrong." I am a good guesser, because I know how to read nonverbal behavior, but I won't play into their defenses. Then there are those who use *joking* or *minimizing* as a defense.

People can use any of these defense mechanisms occasionally and the behavior may be seen as a protective reaction to a particularly stressful situation, not a habitual practice. We look for patterns, behaviors people use consistently. None of these mechanisms works in treatment. They are identified for what they are—behaviors that mask true feelings—first by the counselors and then by the others in treatment.

People develop defense mechanisms to protect themselves when they lack other resources. There's always a payoff, and we have to help them figure out what the payoff is. When it's identified, people often recoil with distaste at finding they exhibit the very behavior they abhor in others, and they work hard to find a more truthful way to present themselves.

ACTIVITIES FOR DAY NINE

Assignment One: Recognizing Defense Mechanisms You Use

This is difficult to do by yourself because you have worked hard building your defense system, and you are reluctant to consider the need for analyzing it. You have invested a lot in your defenses, and you are not going to give them up willingly! I have constructed situations to which hypothetical people respond, using the kinds of defense mechanisms discussed in today's classroom, giving first a sample response, and then the payoff. Make an honest search of your own behavior, and if you identify any of the mechanisms as ones you use, put a check mark by it.

_____ **Blaming**

Johanna failed to pass her licensing exam: "The test was biased. I was distracted because my daughter had smashed the fender of my car. I was coming down with a cold, and the instructor who prepared me for the exam emphasized all the wrong things. No wonder I failed."

Payoff: Johanna doesn't have to face the fact that she didn't study hard enough.

_____ **Projecting**

Ralph's son has trouble making friends. "He doesn't seem to realize that his attitude leaves a lot to be desired.

I tried to teach him how to make friends, but he won't listen. He's stuck-up and is always complaining. I can't imagine how he got that way. I have always been a good influence."

Payoff: By projecting onto his son the very character defects he has, and that his son has learned from him, Ralph doesn't have to examine his own behavior.

_____ Judging

Mona's neighbor's teenage children are in trouble with the law again. She tells another neighbor, "If their mother had stayed at home with those children when they were growing up, they wouldn't be in trouble like this now."

Payoff: Mona feels a sense of moral superiority making this judgment. It also corroborates her own decision to forsake a career to stay home with *her* children when they were growing up, which she now feels too insecure to pursue.

_____ Patronizing

Jim's fiancée is studying to be a lawyer: "She's becoming quite the little grind, just buries that cute nose of hers in the books for days at a time. I tell her at this rate she'll be a better lawyer than I am."

Payoff: By diminishing his fiancée's efforts, Jim increases his status and minimizes the possible threat of career conflict.

_____ Explaining

Maria has an argument with her sister: "I haven't been able to get along with her for years. When we were little, she used to pick on me and she's never stopped. Dad always preferred her, and Mom took my side, so there was never any possibility for us to work out things between ourselves. My sister lives in the past and can't see Dad no longer respects her, because she's just not aware situations change. I think that's because when she was a little kid, she was sick a lot and got shut down. She lives in a dream world."

Payoff: By minutely examining the psychological motives of her sister, Maria can avoid looking at the real reason for the conflict.

_____ Intellectualizing

Rose is lonely: "My inability to make friends stems from a childhood spent with adults who enriched my life greatly, took me to cultural events, read me great literature, and heightened my awareness far beyond the normal capacity of a child. To this day I need to be overstimulated. Only a well-read, well-developed mind is able to keep my interest. I would rather stay home and read great literature than spend time at a party where people talk of trivial things. I put a high value on my mental capacity and am willing to forsake the friendship of others if they can't appreciate it."

Payoff: Rose can avoid the risk of being with people who might surpass her mental capacity. She can stay at home and continue to believe that she is the brightest one she knows.

_____ Generalizing

Al didn't get into the college of his choice: "They never take people from my part of the country. They always want to fill up their enrollment with students from the East or West Coast. I also heard too many people who want to study engineering applied this year. Or maybe it's just that they don't like people of my ethnic persuasion."

Payoff: Al cushions his disappointment by making blanket statements about why he was rejected, thus avoiding having to take it personally.

_____ People-Pleasing

Sandra is running for president of her block association: "I have a hundred phone calls to make today. I'm baking a little something for my next-door neighbor, who's under the weather, and need to drop in on my sister-in-law. She could stand for some cheering up after her accident. Then I told the outgoing president of our group that I'd take care of the mailing, so I have to get to the post office. Two people said they'd help, and they've both canceled. I guess I'll just do it myself. It will save time in the end."

Payoff: By busily doing everyone favors, Sandra can feel important. She can also mask the fact that no one ever does her any favors, because she is so busy doing instead of being.

_____ Withdrawing

Patrick has asked a woman friend to go to a dinner dance and has been turned down: "I really didn't want to go anyway. I hate those affairs. I can put the time to good use by finishing a report this weekend and cleaning the garage. I like being by myself. I'm good company and always spend my time alone productively. Dances and social affairs always end up making me feel like I'm wasting time and money."

Payoff: By not asking someone else, he avoids the pain of further rejection.

_____ Depression

Judith didn't get picked for the vocal competition: "What's the use? I work and work and someone else comes along who doesn't even study voice and gets it. Nothing comes easy for me. Why is it always like that? I've been disappointed so many times, I don't know why I continue to torture myself. The hell with it. I'm through trying to get anywhere. I'm just wasting my time."

Payoff: Judith's defeated attitude protects her from trying further. Feeling sorry for herself is at least some comfort, and the bad mood she's in keeps others away, confirming her worst fears about herself.

_____ Joking

Mary Lou has to buy a new swimsuit because last year's is too small: "Oh, look, a sale on cabana wear. Why don't I just buy the cabana? Remember the tent dress? I might start a new fashion trend."

Payoff: Her friends laugh, and Mary Lou hides her shame at having put on so much weight.

_____ Minimizing

Rosalie got turned down for an appointment she badly wanted: "Oh, it's nothing. I wasn't ready to make any changes anyway. It's not that much of a promotion and the salary differential is peanuts because it would have put me in a new tax bracket. Besides, it's up on a different floor, and I would have had to make all new friends."

Payoff: She saves face with her coworkers and doesn't have to acknowledge her disappointment.

If you checked off less than three defense mechanisms, you have some soul-searching to do. If you checked off six or more, you're working hard. If you checked off more than ten, you might be being a little hard on yourself.

Assignment Two: Down Side

People tend to keep using the same defense systems until they get tired of not getting results or the defenses no longer work. For every payoff there is a loss. What is it about your defense of choice that leaves you dissatisfied? What is its major shortcoming? How do you _feel_ after you have once again resorted to hiding behind your mask while under stress?

Assignment Three: An Alternative Response

Think of the last time you resorted to your defensive response of choice. Write an alternative script for that moment, in which your spirit is given a chance to respond. Imagine that moment without the fear that triggers your defensiveness. Imagine that moment being handled by you without fear, with good sense and respect for yourself.

A DAY IN THE LIFE

Martha   *I had the strangest dream. It was in Technicolor, I swear to God. I just realized I have always dreamed in black and white, or at least don't remember dreaming colors. Those colors were so wonderful! The dream is like pictures—flashes of hollyhocks, bright pink and red and white, and I remember now I used to make ladies out of them. Upside down, their petals made perfect long skirts. And the dream kept going on with these colors and pictures. In one dream I went from flower to flower, like I was flying. And I felt dirt and poured water on it. I walked in the mud. I was at the Catskills. There was a hotel right on the lake we used to go to. Then I am in the water and it is like silk, it is a hot day. The sun is burning my skin. People are laughing on the porch. They start to sing. Now they are dancing. I was dancing too, barefooted between two rows of tomato plants, with big red tomatoes and yellow flowers. It was such a good dream. I feel like crying but I'm happy. Maybe something good is going to happen.*

DAY TEN

Recognizing Defensive Behavior Patterns

Jean, Elaine, and Tony are typical patients who were in treatment at the same time. They all brought with them the particular defensive behaviors they had used much of their lives to protect themselves from getting too close to their real feelings. During the first week of treatment, they used all their defense mechanisms to the hilt, intensifying their behavior because long-buried feelings were beginning to surface.

The behavior patterns they used during that first week are described in the following paragraphs, each with a subheading that defines common defense mechanisms you may be using. Additional mechanisms are italicized:

Blaming

Jean sees her problems as being caused by her jealous and emotionally unstable mother, her dominating and manipulative father, her competitive and people-pleasing sister, and her abusive ex-husband. She is so preoccupied with their faults she can gloss over her own contributions to the endless conflicts in her life. By constantly *creating crisis* she gets lost in the details of the chaos, which protects her from having to look at what's really going on.

Impulsiveness

Jean's impulsiveness drives her from one end of the emotional spectrum to the other. Her moods change from one moment to the next, as well as her opinions of others. Her *promiscuity* is another defense. She relates to others sexually rather than as people as a way of *avoiding intimacy*, which frightens her.

Enmeshing

All her life Jean has been unsure about where she ends and other people begin. Her enmeshment with her family, constantly playing the role assigned to her of Bad Girl, at the same time she tries to win their approval, contributes to her lack of identity. She is involved in a popularity contest among the younger patients and she quickly became the spokesperson for others who want to confront aggressive Gloria about her antisocial behavior. Jean impulsively takes on the role of chief confronter because it is what she has always done.

Analyzing Data

Jean loves to try to make sense of what's happening, but experience and understanding can't happen simultaneously. In order to experience she would just have to be, and that is too threatening for Jean to attempt at this point. Analysis keeps her in her head and her body at bay.

Performing

Because she is so bright and so verbal, people are drawn to her. Her *extremism* and well-developed *humor* make for good storytelling, but they mask what's really happening. Jean's need to be "on," the center of attention, keeps her out of touch with her real feelings.

Rebellion

If Jean can redirect the energy she puts into her combativeness, she will be able to make great strides, but so far she doesn't feel safe enough to drop her defenses as a warrior against injustice and fight her addiction instead. She needs to feel safe to do that, and having never felt that way, she doesn't trust the loving environment she has found herself in. But she wants to. Her lack of passivity is her saving grace.

People-Pleasing

Elaine's major defense mechanism is to keep everybody happy, but no matter how hard she tries, she fails. Her efforts to get close to people like Jean don't succeed because they see her as a phony. She is able to get close only to other people-pleasers, and the intimacy of that contact is shallow because they all have the same objective—to be liked rather than to get to know each other.

Caretaking

By the third day in treatment, Elaine had taken a new patient under her wing. She is constantly on the alert for ways to meet others' needs, and the question she asks most is, "Is there anything I can do?" Her caretaking extends to her husband and daughter at home. She worries that they won't be able to function without her, then gets upset when they can.

Being Nondirect

Elaine is a classic passive–aggressive. She lacks the courage to be confrontational, particularly with her formidable roommate Gloria, and so she gets involved indirectly in other people's affairs. *Piggybacking* is one of the ways she becomes involved, identifying with others who do take action as long as doing so doesn't interfere with her people-pleasing. Her *busyness* keeps her mind off her problems, particularly her family life, which is in a shambles. Her concentration on whether other patients are abiding by the rules and whether she should tell on them fills up her emptiness. *Smiling* keeps others at bay, *forgetting* her home situation makes it easier to smile, and by *numbing her body* she hopes to keep old, fearful feelings from rising.

Although Elaine is full of defenses, she truly wants to find a way out of the dilemma she's in. She desires the peace of mind she has never known, and she is willing to look at her behavior and see it for what it really is, even if it disgusts her.

Denial

Tony, on the other hand, is not willing to look. Of the three patients, he has made the least progress and is still in deep denial. Denial is a way people learn to live in a hostile environment, and Tony's work and family life are certainly that. Although Tony is well liked by the other patients, he is *isolating* himself emotionally. Although he has big problems, he is constantly *minimizing* them. In group therapy he is *playing it safe*, and surprisingly *compliant* for someone who is so aggressive in his professional life. He has learned how to avoid conflict when he doesn't have to confront someone.

In treatment, we work hard at challenging defense structures because you can't bond when you're defensive. Imagine two medieval knights in full armor embracing each other, giving each other's helmet a peck. That's about how close you can get when you haven't let go of your defense mechanisms.

During this second week, as the self-image begins to crack, patients need to look to others to see how they are doing, for they are still convinced the image they have been portraying is their real self. They believe they are defined by what they have achieved, the roles they play in life of wife, husband, son, daughter, student, or employee. How others see them is the only confirmation they feel they have, particularly at a time when they are not sure whether the image they have been projecting is really how the world has seen them after all. In such an insecure time, they find it necessary to hide the feelings, wants, and needs of their real selves, for that identity is still too nebulous to hold on to. Instead, they become intensely involved with how others see them, as if they would disappear without that reference. They are particularly attracted to other addicts, who also believe in the "I am not enough" dictum. With all the deprivations they have been going through—of food and other mood-altering substances, plus their inability to practice their workaholism and relationship addictions—they are intensely devoted to externals.

Inside, the person they really are still feels like a void. They feel empty, fragmented, full of rage and hurt—like little children abandoned by their parents in a room without toys—deprived, helpless, and confused. When they are not feeling the anger and pain of loss of identity, they feel an abyss of nothingness. They are bored, listless, distracted, depressed.

If you feel the same way, rejoice. This stage, painful though it may be, is part of the process you are now engaged in. If you don't allow these feelings to be experienced and expressed, they will intensify to the point where you will have to numb them with food or another substance, creating a little short-term pleasure in exchange for some more long-term pain, and then you'll be back on the roller coaster again, hating all the "downs." If you allow yourself to experience and express these feelings, they will be done with and you can move on. Your need for help at this point may be overwhelming.

If you are not experiencing any feelings, either you don't have an addiction to food or you're kidding yourself. That's just another defense. It may work for a while, but the real you knows better. Keep reading, and remember, the people who are in the most pain are the ones who are numb. Perhaps you should be asking yourself what your numbness is concealing. What could be the source of this pain of yours that is so great you have to shut down all feelings?

Moving from external to internal is a process that involves developing a healthy body image, exercise and good nutrition, boundary development, reality testing, and taking action. By avoiding the comparison of yourself with others, striving for balance and less rigidity, and realizing that perfectionism never leads to happiness, you can keep yourself committed to this process.

It doesn't happen by magic or overnight, the way we addicts like it, but it does happen.

ACTIVITIES FOR DAY TEN

Assignment One

Describe three experiences you have had since last week in which you were aware of using a defensive behavior pattern. What was the reason for your needing to protect yourself? What was the result? Did the defense get you what you wanted?

Assignment Two: You Are a Celebration of Life

To the affirmation of the first week, add this additional line:

> I am not my body.
> I am free.
> I am as God created me.
> I am part of a community.

Assignment Three: Defensive Role Playing

The defensive roles in the following list are common among fearful people with an unclear identity. The quotations are typical responses to help you identify them. Which of the roles do you play? What are the advantages and disadvantages of each? When do you find it necessary to assume the role? Examine the fear that motivates it. What would happen if you didn't need to play these roles?

1. SUPERMAN   "I know what to do."
   WONDER WOMAN

2. PERFECT PETER	"Of course I always do it right. What is the problem?"
3. PLEASING POLLY	"I want to make you happy."
4. BLAMING BETTY BITCHING BILL	"Why can't you do it right?"
5. FIXING FANNY MOTHER HUBBARD	"I will take care of it."
6. PAUL THE PROPHET NEGATIVE NAN	"It will never work anyway."
7. WHO-CARES WILLIE NEVER-MIND NELLY	"It does not matter."
8. CHARLIE THE COMPUTER FAMILY PLANNER	"What do you want to do next summer?"
9. OPPOSITE ORVILLE PARTY-POOPER PEARL	"Be careful jogging. It could become an addiction."
10. RUN-ABOUT RUTH HURRY HARRY	"I have to run."
11. DEACON DAN	"I will tell you what is wrong with this country, etc., etc."
12. LOGICAL LARRY	"It does not make sense."
13. ORPHAN ANNIE	"I do not know why all these things happen to me."

14. WONDERFUL WIZARD	"Gosh, everything is fantastic."
15. CHIEF GURU	"Just stay calm."
16. SLAVING SYLVIA	"I never have time for anything but work."
17. MARGARET MARTYR	"I guess I deserve it."
18. FUNNY FRANK	"Did you ever hear the story . . ."
19. QUIET QUIGLEY	"I don't know."
20. FRANTIC FRANNIE	"Oh, my God! What do we do now?"
21. TERRIBLE TERRY	"This is the worst town I have ever lived in."

A DAY IN THE LIFE

Jenny *My roommate Martha is really driving me nuts and I can't—I don't—say anything. Why? She has to control everything. The towels have to be folded exactly her way, and the shampoo and conditioner bottles have to be just so in the bathroom. She opens and shuts the curtains a hundred times a day—she even tries to control the sunlight! She talks a blue streak, even when I am obviously reading a book or writing. She complains about everything. She sees herself as a woman of wisdom but doesn't have a clue that others see her as a pest.*

Two P.M. A good thing has happened. Unassertive I actually got up the nerve to request a roommate change. Instead I meet Peggy, who is moving in today to become my third roommate. I like her a lot. She is very sick, though. She's been bulimic for ten years. Martha is busy giving her nutritional advice and reeling off her House Rules (the list gets longer every day) and Peggy just totally ignores her. At one point she looked her straight in the eye and said, "Oh, buzz off. I've got things on my mind." Martha's jaw dropped a mile and instead of getting mad she just sort of sank into herself. I felt kind of bad for her.

I just had a session with Bob. He says I'm too focused on other people—how I feel about them rather than how I am feeling about myself and my issues. I keep telling him I don't have any issues, just lifelong depression. What can I bring up to get upset about? That my parents got divorced? Big deal. That I have unsuccessful love affairs with married men? So what else is new? I just feel so empty. It's like there's something bottled up inside me that can't find the way out. I haven't found that way out yet. Oh, how I want to get out of this jam! I really want to get better and am so frustrated that I'm stuck.

•

DAY ELEVEN

Types of Communication

There are four basic types of communication: aggressive, passive, passive–aggressive, and assertive. Only assertive behavior truly communicates. The other forms rise out of hostility and fear, and they rarely work. Just because people use a particular behavior doesn't mean they *are* that behavior. They are free at any time to choose another style that will get them what they really want, but they have to discover what that behavior is before they can change it.

Aggressive

Aggressive types use threatening, accusing, fighting, and attacking behavior because they feel angry and frustrated. Much of the time they express themselves like little children, explosively, impulsively, and uncontrollably. They are demanding, dominating, and quick to blame and put down others. Rarely do they see themselves as aggressors. In fact, they often see themselves as victims! Unfortunately, their style of communication will only result in more anger and frustration, as others tend to dislike and avoid them. Aggressive people act under the misconception that they have the right to get what they want no matter the cost to someone else. They suffer from an "I" complex and see themselves as the center of the universe. The term "King Baby" often fits them perfectly. Their perception of the world is that someone has to win (themselves, of course) and someone else has to lose. Unless they are in the dominant position, they are so threatened they can't communicate, and their bottom line, "My way or the highway," makes compromise all but impossible.

It is difficult to get aggressive types to examine their behavior, and when they do see the truth about themselves, they are likely to respond with more anger and frustration because it is the only thing they know. Win—lose is their objective.

Passive

Passive behavior is acting in a manner that allows other people to get what they want at the passive person's expense. Like the aggressive style, it is the behavior of little children: helpless, receptive, enduring what others impose without resistance. Whereas aggressors act like tyrannical two-year-olds, passive people act like infants. Their perception of the world is that somehow, somewhere, someone other than themselves will act responsibly and rescue them from the dilemma they're in.

A person who uses passive behavior quite naturally feels out of control and uses the behavior as an indirect way to control others. Underneath the placid surface is a lot of rage, and with the same lack of control that characterizes the behavior, the passive person will suddenly turn aggressive in a vain effort to regain control. The result is a lack of respect, from others and for oneself, and constant frustration. Passive people are an energy drain. People don't want to associate with victims, almost as if such behavior were contagious, and the passive person's inability to attract others only feeds into his or her feelings of worthlessness. Aggressives are full of contempt for passive people's inability to take risks and seek them out for combat, for the passive person fits perfectly into their "I win—you lose" scenario.

Passive–Aggressive

More common than either passive or aggressive behavior is a combination of the two. Because it appears to be adult behavior, it is more socially acceptable. Passive–aggressive behavior is an indirect expression of hostility, resisting authority and controlling others, and it is much harder to detect, in oneself or in others, because it is childlike behavior in disguise. Anger and helplessness combine to take the form of clever sarcasm or unkind words, procrastination and dawdling, inefficiency or forgetfulness. Passive–aggressive types are the backstabbers, the ones who say, "Don't tell a soul but . . . ." They are the ones who agree to do something and then come up with a last-minute excuse and leave you dangling. Devious and manipulating, they lose even when they win because they don't know whether they've won fair and square or because they've manipulated the results. Indirect to the extreme, they punish others by punishing themselves. Passive–aggressives like to seek out passive placators who don't think their ideas or feelings are worth defending, then walk all over them, hating the passivity they recognize, if not acknowledge, within themselves. They will also placate aggressive people and then seek to undermine them. I heard a definition recently from Robert Subby: Passive–aggressive is when a dog puts his paw on your shoulder, pisses on your leg, and licks your face at the same time!

Assertive

Whereas the other types of communication are defenses, often automatic in nature, that rarely get people what they want, assertiveness is a learned behavior that provides at the very least a feeling of respect, if not the desired results. It's a general observation of mine that people will treat you with the same amount of respect as you command. No one ever gets it by pitiful pleading or an uproar. Only those whose behavior is a role model for respect will get it from others.

Assertive behavior is respectful of the rights of others. It is honest, direct, and firm. It makes self-expressive statements rather than asking questions. Assertive people think enough of themselves to express their thoughts and feelings without expecting others to agree with them. They have no need to control the responses of others, but they do need to be understood. They may not get what they want, but at least they're clear about what it is.

Nonassertive people confuse the goal of being liked with being respected. They have learned to act in inferior ways because they believe they *are* inferior, and that the rights of others are more important than their own. They are self-conscious before superior and authority figures. They are easily hurt by what others say and do. Their greatest fear is that they may offend. In their evasiveness, they often offend anyway, especially themselves, by constantly abnegating their own beliefs and desires and allowing others to maneuver them into situations they don't want to be in. To minimize their discomfort, they limit their experiences and don't use their full potential.

Assertive people respect themselves and others enough to tell the truth. They feel free to reveal themselves: "This is me. This is what I feel, think, and want." They can communicate with people on all levels—authority figures, strangers, friends, family, little children—with the same open, direct, honest, and appropriate manner. Their personalities do not change, chameleonlike, depending upon whom they are talking to. They enjoy the comfort that comes simply with being. They have an active orientation to life and go after what they want rather than what others tell them they should want. In contrast to the passive person who waits for things to happen, assertive people have the courage to go out and make things happen for themselves, and they enjoy the feeling of power that comes from growing up emotionally as well as intellectually, knowing they don't have to act like helpless children in order to get by in the world. Aware they can't always win, they gracefully accept their limitations and do not try to force their will on others. They strive in spite of the odds to make a good try, so whether they get their way or not, they maintain their self-respect. That's a win–win situation.

The difference between assertive and all other kinds of behavior is a combination of courage and respect. Aggressive people have no trouble finding the courage to say what's on their minds, but they lack respect for others. Passive people have too much respect for the opinion of others and lack the courage to express their own. Like the Cowardly Lion, the Tin Man, and the Scarecrow in *The Wizard of Oz*, each type of communication other than assertive lacks a quality that prevents a person practicing it from being whole and functional.

Hardly anyone is assertive by nature, and it is a behavior rarely found in a person who grew up in a dysfunctional family where mixed messages were the norm. Assertive behavior is most often a learned skill.

It is acting in a manner that allows a person to obtain what he or she wants while not violating the rights of others. That may seem like a tightrope act at first, but the insecurity will vanish with practice. Once you become comfortable in your new behavior, it will be infinitely better than the styles you have been using, which either allowed people to walk all over you or drove them away or made them confused, while it gave you feelings of discomfort that arose when you knew you were not being true to yourself.

Imagine this situation: You are standing in a supermarket line and someone cuts in front of you. An aggressive person responds by making a scene—"How *dare* you!"—which often backfires. Others in line are offended more by the outburst than the original indiscretion and separate themselves from the aggressor. Sympathy may actually be generated for the trespasser because of the violence of the response. Passive people, on the other hand, are not fully convinced the offender doesn't have the right to usurp their place in line, and even if they do feel they have the right to protest, they are afraid to offend or ruffle feathers. Maintaining the peace is always their first objective. Meanwhile, they seethe inwardly, thinking of all the times they have felt helpless in the face of aggression.

Passive–aggressive people roll their eyes at others in line, murmuring under their breath about how "Some people have such nerve" and "Who do they think they are?" but never directly confront the offender. They may feel some relief in the approval of others, but never justice, and their indirect form of communication, talking behind someone's back, is an indication to others that they can't be trusted.

The assertive person confronts the offender in a quiet but firm voice: "When you cut in line in front of me, I feel very angry." If the offender says, "So what? I don't care," assertive people are ready to plan a course of action and stick to it: "And if you don't go to the end of the line, I will talk to the manager." Assertive people don't need the support of others in the line, although they will often find they have their respect for being able to voice what the others may lack the courage to say, but winning a popularity contest is not the objective of the assertive person. Establishing and defending boundaries is. Even if the manager can't be found and the obnoxious line-cutter sails out of the supermarket without a reprimand, assertive people have the satisfaction of knowing they were true to themselves, worthy of protest. A lot of life's little inequities take place in situations similar to the supermarket line. People who fail to act assertively can put themselves into emotional tempests over these small infractions of the rules of good behavior, and their tranquillity can be disturbed for hours afterward. Because the infractions are minor and caused by strangers, such situations are a good place to practice assertive behavior. It's easier to confront a stranger than a significant person in your life, and each situation in which you act assertively—in spite of the fear and misgivings you may feel—will give you the courage to change your behavior when it really counts.

ACTIVITIES FOR DAY ELEVEN

Assignment One: Your Habitual Communication Style

What is your habitual communication style: aggressive, passive, or passive–aggressive? Describe the last time you used it. Imagine you could go back to that moment. Describe how you could have responded assertively.

Assignment Two: Your Nonhabitual Communication Style

Take two socks and create hand puppets out of them by stuffing a little tissue into each toe to represent the heads. Identify one of the puppets as yourself and the other as a significant person in your life with whom you are in conflict. Make features and hair for each puppet with felt tip markers, yarn, buttons, or bits of fabric.

I have found I can tell people what's really on my mind, and they can really hear me if I communicate from my core being. It's amazing how direct you can be as long as you speak from your inner self. In this exercise you will recreate a moment of conflict and replay it with intention and calmness, acknowledging who you really are.

Choose a recent conflict, script it as if you were writing a scene in a play, and then perform it in two different versions with your hand puppets. The first time portray the conflict as it actually happened, with both people using their habitual communication style.

When the conflict scene is written and played out verbatim, be prepared for the emergence of a lot of feelings. That's why this activity is a private one. You can be in the eye of the hurricane and move as slowly and carefully as you need to, from word to word.

The second time, rewrite just your lines in the script using an assertive communication style that feels right to you. Actually writing the words gives you time to edit—time we never get in real life but which you will serve you well the next time your feelings are out of control and you can't think straight.

Here is an example: A mother and daughter are deeply enmeshed. The mother's guilt for neglecting her daughter as a child has resulted in an overly generous response to her as an adult. She gives her too much in terms of loans and favors, and then resents how little she has left for herself and how little her daughter gives back. In that way she is rescripting the scenario of thirty years ago when she was a young unmarried mother with an infant, only this time instead of being neglectful, she is being generous to the point of sainthood.

The daughter, on the other hand, both resents and takes advantage of her mother's generosity. She knows it comes from guilt rather than true affection and is angry over that. She doesn't trust her mother, for when long-term unexpressed anger finally erupts, it is always cruel and hurtful in the way only family members know how to wound.

A recent conflict was over an unreturned book. It began innocently enough with the mother asking a bit too sweetly, "Oh and by the way, whatever happened to that book I loaned you?" Because the lost book had special meaning, she soon flew into a rage over the item the daughter had borrowed and not returned. The daughter flew into an even greater rage, going through the litany of her mother's neglect and how she had ripped the daughter off her entire life. With a loud slam of the door and the parting words, "And I won't take care of you in your old age," the conflict ended, with the mother in a shambles of guilt, rage, and grief, and the daughter feeling quite righteous and vindicated. Neither was able to resolve the conflict, and it still affects their lives in a hurtful way.

When the mother–daughter conflict is rescripted, the mother becomes focused on the book and the book alone. She decides there are other more appropriate forums for the expression of her accumulated pent-up feelings. This particular incident is about an unreturned book, not years of resentment. In the rescripted scene the mother's parting line becomes, "Do you think you could replace it? There are book-finding stores that do that." When she plays out the daughter's parting shot of "And I won't take care of you in your old age," the mother bursts into gales of laughter. The conflict goes from tragedy to comedy. What can't be resolved in anger often *can* be resolved through laughter, as long as we never forget to laugh at ourselves.

After you have performed your two little plays, write a critique about the drama as if you had been in the audience looking on, with speculations on a hopeful resolution.

A DAY IN THE LIFE

Chuck   *Something is happening to me that I can't explain, only feel. I feel so good! Yet nothing I would exactly define as "good" has happened to me that I should feel this way. My wife was the first to notice, over the phone. She said, "What are you so happy about?" and I said, "Gee, I don't know." She said, "Well, you sound different somehow." I wanted to know exactly what she meant because she was sounding sort of accusatory, like I was in the hospital and shouldn't be feeling so good. She said my voice had changed, like something was lifted, this little worried quality, a tension, that she hadn't even noticed was there until it was gone. I said to her, "Jeannie, I think I know what's different. I have come to the realization that I can just be Chuck—not Chuck the Good Guy— and the worried sound that's always been in my voice was about never being enough, no matter how much weight I gained. I always had to be Chuck the Good Guy, or Chuck to the Rescue. The truth is, I didn't even know just plain Chuck. Now that I've met him, I don't need to have to be anybody else."*

The other thing that's making me feel so good is this rage that I let go in group. I sat both my parents in the empty chairs and let them have it. I couldn't get angry with my body, though, the way they want us to here. Violence was my parents' way; I used my words. I raged and roared about what had happened to their children because of their alcoholism—to me, to my kid brother

Harry who can't have a relationship that lasts more than a year, and to Sally, who just can't seem to get it together. But my rage really came when Bob the therapist told me to focus on what they had done to me. I was so angry at him for that—how dare he! I kept thinking. I've never known such rage. It went through me like white lightning. Bob had challenged my deepest belief—that I didn't matter. I felt like I was coming apart. It was so hard to let go of this belief that had kept me together all these years—that it didn't matter what was done to me as long as I could protect everyone else. But then everybody—Jenny and Martha and Laurie and Gordon and Bob—put their arms around me and supported me. I could feel their energy vibrating around me and their love enclosing me. I felt like a helpless baby chick and they were the mother. I cried so hard I had to sit down. I felt from them the love and caring I couldn't feel for myself. I will never forget that circle of people and how they allowed me to bring out of hiding this little kid, Chuckie. I can see him now, with his missing front tooth. I can see the look in his eyes as he prays for the fighting to stop. I can do for him what wasn't done for me. I can take him out of that place where he's been hiding, that bad place where I didn't know I left him a long time ago. I can take this little kid, famished for love and affection, and I can take him out to play. I can take him to the playground and we can swing, and fool around on the monkey bars. I can pitch to him until he gets good at connecting with a bat, and then he can pitch to me. There was no place in this world for Chuckie before I came here, and the surprise of meeting him here was the last thing I expected.

DAY TWELVE

Expressing Feelings

Feelings are neither good nor bad. They just are. They're what we have the most of and know the least about. We can't control having them, but we can change them by modifying the way we respond to them. We can channel them into action, not reaction.

Now that we have learned to identify and validate all those feelings we have been denying and medicating with food, what do we do with them? How can they be expressed to our advantage? Most likely, the old pattern has been a long simmer followed by a sudden outburst, which inevitably backfires and never gets us what we want. After feeling victimized for so long, when we finally express ourselves, we become the victimizer! Then, full of remorse and guilt, we go back into our shell and decide we are hopeless communicators.

There is hope. It lies in learning an entirely new mode of expression. We need to develop a new syntactical structure that will contain our feelings and still allow for thought. It is simple and involves six small words: "When you," "I feel," and "I need."

When You . . .

Here is a hypothetical situtation: Your mother interrupts you for the twenty-fourth time in a telephone conversation. Your stomach is churning over the memory of years and years of enduring her interruptions, for all the times you have remained silent, for all the other indignities you have suffered because she doesn't listen to you, seemingly doesn't care what you have to say, doesn't want to hear about your hopes, dreams, fears, and ideas. After you hang up the telephone, you decide you will punish her by not calling her for a while. Weeks later, she calls you and berates you for neglecting her. You explode.

That's the old pattern.

Here is the new way you can express your feelings. You can practice it the next time someone who is significant to your life and purports to care about you says or does something that elicits hurt feelings. Note I didn't say "makes you feel bad" or "causes you pain." "Elicit" means to call up, to evoke, to draw forth, to bring up something potential or latent. Merely the voice tones of a significant person in your life can hit a childhood memory trace and put you back into the child state. The action of the other person has caused those feelings *that are already there* to emerge and be reexperienced.

As soon as you say "you" the other person will get defensive. When you respond by saying, "You make me feel bad," the other person has every reason to say, "What did I do that was so bad? You're always overreacting." Short of physical violence, another person can't "make" you feel bad. If the person interrupting you was someone you didn't care about or who had no emotional hold over you, you might be annoyed or simply tell yourself not to seek out that person's company anymore. But it's your mother, and you're in turmoil, a seething mass of feelings. You care!

Begin your response by taking a deep breath and then letting it out. When people are in a "feeling state" they often forget to breathe. They take a sharp intake of breath and then hold it, under some kind of delusion that they are controlling themselves. This is no time to deny oxygen to your brain. Breathing also gives you time to collect your thoughts.

The first phase begins with the words "When you" and ends with an action: "When you interrupt me," "When you raise your voice," "When you give me unsolicited advice," "When you are late," "When you forget," "When you criticize me," "When you leave a mess in the kitchen"—whatever the present action is. Keep it to the incident that brought up the feelings, not all the other times it happened. "You always" and "You never" shut down communication and leave room for debate. Avoid extreme statements and stick to the present.

I Feel . . .

The second phase is to learn to confront others by saying "I feel." You can't be condemned for having feelings. They're yours and you have a right to them.

What *do* you feel? Angry? Insignificant? Humiliated? Afraid? Annoyed? Check the list of "feeling words" from the Activities for Day Five if you're having difficulty identifying exactly what you're feeling.

Maybe the other person will respond, "I don't think your feelings are well-founded. You shouldn't feel that way." The response to that is, "But I do."

Notice that the statement "I feel" does not talk about "you." Avoid that word and you will be amazed how often people will be able to hear you out. As soon as you start making "you" accusations, the other party is ready for a fight. Talking about yourself and your feelings disarms them. Instead of saying "When you don't listen to me, you make me so mad," say "When you turn on the TV while I'm talking to you, I feel ignored."

"But" negates whatever is stated prior to it, such as "I know you don't intend to be rude, but" or "You may not know this bothers me, but." That word crops up in communication all the time, and it's usually meant to soften the blow. Instead it gets in the way of communication.

You may find that your respectful statement of feelings produces no response at all, or wordless surprise or confusion at what to say. Into that silence you can inject the third part of the response.

I Need . . .

Rather than say "If only you would . . ." speak of your desires. It's disrespectful to say you want someone to change. Instead, express what you need from that person.

What *do* you need? Maybe you have never thought much about that before: "I need respect for my decisions." "I need someone to listen to me." "I need help." "I need understanding."

Making a simple statement about what you need moves the communication forward. Instead of veering toward accusation and blame, plus a round of nit-picking debate about the incident that provoked the confrontation, stating what you need offers a solution. You have given the person who has offended you a graceful way out of the confrontation, if he or she wants to take it. If not, what does that say about the person? It may be painful to realize that someone who means something to you isn't interested in meeting your needs, but it's better to know than to guess, and you have really cleared the air by your declaration.

You may not get what you want when you express your feelings, but you will feel powerful afterward. You have been honest, open, and direct. You will have respected yourself and other people enough to tell them what's going on with you. People will treat you with the same amount of respect as you command: you have been the role model for what you expect to get back, whether you get it or not.

Most of all, you will not have made a fool of yourself by sputtering and fuming, and then enduring the usual backlash. You will feel confident that you can communicate your feelings and needs again and again, and you will feel released from the terrible prison in which you struggle with your feelings and never get them expressed to the outside world in a way that gets heard. Congratulations!

ACTIVITIES FOR DAY TWELVE

Assignment One: When you . . . I feel . . . I need . . .

Recall the last time you either failed to express your feelings or botched the job with a significant person in your life—a spouse, lover, son or daughter, parent, friend, or neighbor. Focus on that situation now, and try to recall the exact words or actions that set you off. Write down what happened here: _____

_____

Now write the response you could have made or will make the next time this situation occurs, beginning with the words "When you": _____

_____

Add the words "I feel" and describe your feelings:

_____

Now add the statement, "I need": _____

_____

How do you feel about the statement you have just made? _____

_____

Assignment Two: Commitment

Make a commitment to yourself here that you will use this new way of expressing your feelings with this significant person in your life the next time it is appropriate to do so.

Assignment Three: The Real Meaning of Stress

Many people find it stressful to express their true feelings and needs, and doing so leaves them feeling bad about themselves. The word "stress" implies that we are under attack from outside sources, and if we could retreat to a mountaintop or beach, our stress would all go away. But the real stress comes from inside, and that's why it always comes with you to the beach or the mountains. When people say they are feeling stressed, they are really feeling guilty, angry, or fearful. Anger is a secondary emotion, experienced as strength, while fear and guilt are experienced as weakness. Many choose anger as a form of expression instead of fear or guilt. Anger is always about something else. In its unexpressed form it becomes resentment, a luxury no addict can afford.

Rather than learn a new relaxation technique, we need to learn how to discharge our anger and get to what's really bothering us. If you could attack the real source of stress in your life, whatever is eating you from the inside, what would that source be? Write in your diary about the fear that can always be found cowering behind your mask of anger. Focus on that cowering person. Why are your shoulders hunched like that? What is buried behind your mask of anger, still causing you difficulty after so many years?

The next time you tell someone "I need . . ." or "I feel . . ." pay attention to the way you feel afterward. If you don't feel good about expressing your true self, something is definitely eating you. It is your responsibility to yourself to find out what that something is, so you can live without the stress those buried feelings are causing you.

Assignment Four: Fear with Action

When you really want to communicate with someone, ask for what you need. Most likely you have trouble doing that, or even knowing what it is you need because you put a low value on giving yourself what you readily give to others. The best way to discover what you need is to look at what you fear, which is usually more readily identifiable. Once you identify your fears, you can know what your needs are, because they are the opposite of your fears. If you fear rejection, you need acceptance. If you fear being controlled, you need autonomy. If you fear abandonment, you need belonging. If you fear being abused, you need nurturance.

> F—False
> E—Evidence
> A—Appearing
> R—Real

Draw a vertical line down the center of a sheet of paper. On the left side write the heading "What I fear" and on the right side, "What I need." In the left column write your three greatest fears. In the right column, write the opposite of each fear and three ways for each that you can give yourself what you need.

You have two choices in giving yourself what you need: fear with action or fear with no action. Choose fear with action because it keeps you moving, whereas fear with no action bogs you down. Fear is never going to leave your life. It's an emotion like love or sadness. You're not doing anything wrong if you're afraid. It's the inaction that's debilitating.

The more you operate out of fear, the greater the likelihood that your fears will come true, for the mind tends to move toward its most dominant thought. The greater your fear of rejection, the more likely you will be rejected and reject others before they have a chance to reject you. If instead you honor your need for acceptance, learn to ask for it, and create situations in which it will likely come about, your needs will take precedence over your fears. Like two ends of a seesaw, the higher the need reaches toward fulfillment, the lower the fear recedes.

You may feel foolish at first asking for what you need, but you will find it disarms people because it is nonconfrontational. It makes you human, because you acknowledge you have needs and are willing to expose your vulnerability. Needs can't be denied, rejected, or argued about. They are a solid basis for honest communication.

A DAY IN THE LIFE

Jenny   Something happened in group today that I have to write down. Martha is working hard there. She is really courageous. What I saw today just tore me apart, the way she cried in that young girl voice, the way she turned into an innocent and awkward thirteen-year-old in front of my eyes. Incest again, her rich uncle. I just can't identify. It's beyond me. My father would never. It's unimaginable. He always treated me with such respect, and his hugs have always been stiff, like he was a stranger. That used to bother me but no more! I feel like these incest victims are completely different from me. They have been places I can't and don't want to imagine. But bad as that place is, at least it's something to find. I can't find anything to work on. I sit there in group day after day just feeling lost. But today as I watched Martha go through all that pain, I realized I have been focused on my irritation with her rather than working on my own stuff.

Four P.M.   I'm supposed to look at the patterns of my choices—the men I pick out to love. First pattern: When I fall in love, it's instant—I mean like fall. The guy then becomes an obsession and I have to marry him and have his babies, all in one week. Second, he always has to be basically unavailable, although I don't necessarily know how unavailable when I first meet him. Roger was married and had two kids. Mike is married and has no kids. Is that progress?

DAY THIRTEEN

Social Skills

Today I want you to feel as if you're back in kindergarten, because we are going to discuss the most elementary matter: social skills—what children are taught when they first go to school and interact with their peers. If you balk at having to focus on such simple matters, may I remind you once again that addiction is a disease of isolation. Focusing on social skills is as appropriate to treating addiction as aspirin is to treating a fever.

Sometimes social skills were never learned, or have been forgotten. A lack of social skills is magnified in adolescence, when the onset of sexuality makes life even more complicated. Hardly anyone gets through that difficult phase of life unscathed, and many of us still feel like adolescents when we enter a room full of strangers at a party, or wait for our first dinner guests to arrive.

Why should it be so hard to be a social being? I say, it's not. In fact, it's so easy it's laughable! To be at ease, all you have to do is put others at ease, look them in the eye, listen to what they say, tell them what's on your mind, and lo and behold—a conversation! Add to that a little laughter, a few hugs, and you've got social skills.

Names

You meet someone new and are introduced. Did you catch the name? No? Why? Was your mind filled with other things, like the impression you were making or what you were going to say? Most people love to hear their own names and feel highly complimented when others remember them. Catching a name during an introduction is simply a matter of practice. Rather than being nervous about what to think or say, concentrate on the moment, for the only thing of importance in it is hearing the person's name. Quiet your mind and listen for it. If you don't catch it, ask for it to be repeated (people usually don't mind doing that at all), and then use it yourself when you reply: "How do you do, Maggie. My name is Janet." If you vocalize the name, your mind registers it much more firmly than if you merely try to register it mentally.

Eye Contact

With the name clearly in mind, look the person in the eyes. What color are they? What do you see in them? Does he or she look away? Eye contact is the most telling form of communication. You can learn much about what strangers are like merely by watching their eyes, as well as being aware of your own.

Because eye contact is learned from our parents, messages can get complicated and even distorted. On the one hand, children are rarely satisfied that they have the parent's attention until they get eye contact. Every parent knows that if two children are crying, the one who stops first is the one who gets the eye contact. On the other hand, parents may never give their children their full attention unless they are angry. How many times have you heard the phrase, spoken in outrage, "Look at me when I talk to you!" That's a negative form of reinforcement, and many children who have heard it from their parents while growing up make eye contact only when they fight. A lot of people actually have to look away to express their feelings and their deeper thoughts.

You can tell a lot about what feelings and thoughts people are having by watching what their eyes are doing. Looking up and to the right means they are trying to remember or put together an image or a picture. Looking up and to the left means they're trying to construct a picture or an image. Looking down and to the right is about attaching feeling to something. Looking down and to the left is about internal dialogue. Usually when people are feeling bad about themselves that's how I can tell. I know they're listening to the dialogues they're having with themselves.

If the eyes are at eye level and they look to the right, they're getting in touch with something they've heard before, such as trying to remember the words of a song. If they're looking eye level and then to the left, they're trying to construct a sound, as my son does when he's trying to write music. There's so much being communicated by eye contact. Much of it we know inside, but we don't *know* that we know.

If you want to establish real intimacy with people, look into their eyes when you talk to them, and look into their eyes when you listen to them. Don't stare or you'll spook them, but if you are truly in search of being "real" with people, they will respond. In fact, they will open up and tell you things that are meaningful to them. Conversations will suddenly be easy because you won't be having to search for superficialities. People are yearning to get beneath the surface of things. Give them half a chance, and they'll be grateful for it.

Voice Image

Anorexics have a special problem with voice image and speak in a tiny, childlike voice. When they say they can't understand why everyone treats them like a child, I say, "Because you speak like a child." Their voices come out of the top of their throats rather than being resonated from the mouth, throat, and chest. No one wants to strain to listen. The metaphor of anorexia is a desire to disappear, and this includes vocally. Making an effort to be heard will diminish the power of that metaphor, and the encouraging feedback received from others will encourage the anorexic to reappear.

Touching

In this dangerous age we live in, physical contact has become far less acceptable than in previous decades. Yet, people still yearn for closeness, and there are many ways to touch that demonstrate caring in a nonthreatening way. The safest place to touch someone is on the forearm. Its close proximity to the fingers, which deal with expression of thought rather than sexuality, makes it a safe place to make physical contact. To most people a touch on the forearm means emphasis, either in understanding or in reply to what has just been said.

Many females, however, feel violated if a man touches them on the upper arm, particularly if it is bare. I think the reason is a lot of women hide their breasts by crossing their arms, and touching the upper arm is tantamount to touching their breasts. If you don't want to offend a woman you've just met, touch her on the forearm. The shoulder is also an inoffensive place to touch. I have found in therapy sessions that if I touch someone on the stomach, all of a sudden they'll start expressing feelings. It's interesting to me that the stomach is the closest to food.

Hugs

A lot of people don't know how to give a proper hug. To me the best hug is eye contact first, to register intimacy, then a simple and spontaneous embrace with body contact coupled with loving thoughts. Pats on the back are for burping babies. The A-frame hug, with lots of space between the bodies, is a half-hearted affair. Then there's the "right boob, left boob" hug. Men have a tendency to hug that way, especially tall men. It's probably a variation of the embrace that features a peck on both cheeks. To me it's a busy hug, and too complicated. Why not just stand still and enjoy it?

In my years of therapy I've found it's the rare person

who doesn't like to be hugged, and that person is inevitably the one who needs it the most. At the center, I don't give hugs just for shakes. I think some people have to be direct and ask for hugs, because that's one of the things people need to learn—to start going after what they want—but if I want to hug spontaneously, I feel free to do so.

It may seem simplistic to you at this point to say that developing social skills will make the difference between relapse and recovery, but I am convinced the reason my treatment program is so successful is that we send people out into the world knowing how to be social beings. People can go into treatment and successfully lose or gain weight, but what difference does that make if they go back out into society still feeling cold and numb and isolated, unable to communicate with others in a meaningful way? Real recovery is about changing life-styles. Practicing basic social skills will do more for your future happiness than any calorie counter, and it's a lot more fun.

ACTIVITIES FOR DAY THIRTEEN

Assignment One: Draw Your Family Tree

Label each member of your family and give each of them a grade that evaluates their social skills. High grades mean they had many close friends and long-term relationships, and that those social skills were passed on to you. Low grades mean few friends and long-term relationships. Write a few paragraphs about what you have learned about your family from doing this exercise and how they influenced your ability to communicate with intimacy.

Assignment Two: Meditation Exercise

Meditation is an important part of Janet Greeson's "Your Life Matters." When people begin to abstain from their compulsive eating patterns, the pain that that coping mechanism had been masking begins to rise. Meditation is a spiritual alternative for dealing with the discomfort of those feelings.

Pain is a necessary part of change, but suffering is optional. As people experience the pain that comes with abstinence, they want to react to it, as that is what they have always done in the past. Reaction to pain is called suffering. Meditation is an alternative coping mechanism that allows the uncomfortable feelings to flow out of you without your resistance, thereby eliminating the need to suffer. Disengaging yourself from the pain of those percolating feelings takes away their power and the resulting suffering that has driven you to compulsive eating.

Early in your abstinence, when you feel overwhelmed with a sense of discomfort—a diffuse, all-encompassing dread, a feeling that life can't go on—it means the emotions you had been burying deep in your unconscious are beginning to rise. Later they will become more specific, but for now they are not truly observable and can be regarded as negative energy that needs to be discharged. Meditation is the conductor of that energy, allowing it to leave you while safely grounding you in a state of awareness in which you remain apart from the feelings, claiming them but not engaging them. It is a purifying process that will soon seem effortless.

The time to meditate is every time the compulsion to return to your destructive eating patterns returns. That compulsion may leave you in as little as a few minutes if you are able to quiet your mind. It is also a good idea to meditate at a certain time each day, such as early in the morning, during breaks in your working day, or in the evening. You don't need to spend more than a few minutes meditating. Five minutes will seem long in the beginning. Later you will find fifteen minutes and eventually a half hour passing without your being aware of time.

"Prayer is when we speak; meditation is when we listen." It's that simple. Meditation doesn't have to be mystical or ritualistic. It merely ceases the endless debates that go on in your head and allows you to be at one with yourself. It helps you escape the boundaries of noise and confusion and puts you on a new plane. In deep meditation you exist simultaneously at different levels of consciousness. Scientists have no way of explaining how a person can be in two different places at the same time, but people who practice meditation don't need an explanation. They feel it. What they are feeling is an increase in serotonin, the "feel good" hormone in the brain.

When people first start to meditate, they are often frustrated because they really become aware of the board meetings going on in their heads. They're supposed to be the chairman of that board, but they seem to have no control over the conversations and the confusion. You can stop all the chatter by focusing on your breathing:

Fill your lungs deeply, using your diaphragm muscles, taking in air to a slow count of eight or ten, and then releasing it all at once—let it go without holding it back. As you let it out, direct the air to where the chatter is and blow it away. When thoughts come into your mind, let them pass without resistance. Don't get frustrated when these thoughts resurface. It's your mind's job to think, and thoughts never stop; they just don't have to be owned. Listen not to them but to the silence in the background, for a message that has yet to come. Soon your thoughts will become the background, just another environmental irritant to ignore, and you will sink to another level of consciousness where you become quiet and at peace.

You will learn to love this state of mind, and to want to repeat the experience. In later exercises you will be given specific tasks to perform while meditating, visualizations that will lead you deeper and deeper into this altered state of consciousness. For today, just enjoy the silence. Set five minutes as your goal, and repeat those five minutes several times throughout the day.

Assignment Three: The Listening Ladder

The goal of listening is understanding. It is the best gift you can give to anyone, and perhaps the best way to communicate love and respect. The next time you have an opportunity to give this gift, remember the following points:

The Listening Ladder

L: Look at the person speaking
A: Ask questions for clarification
D: Don't change the subject
D: Don't interrupt
E: Express emotions with control
R: Responsibility to listen

You, as a good listener, look into the eyes of whomever is speaking and see that person for whom he or she is today, not someone he or she reminds you of. You devote your energy to taking in what the speaker has to say, withholding evaluation of the message and not judging it or overreacting to it. The good listener in you does not interrupt or change the subject, but when feedback is requested, you will give it, clearly and sincerely. You are tolerant and don't let a person's manner of speaking turn you off. You concentrate on facts but listen for the feelings behind what is being said, and you don't let emotion-arousing words disrupt the listening process. If someone is having difficulty expressing emotion, lean back. If someone is really desperate to be heard, lean forward. Responsibility for listening also means letting people know if you don't have time to listen rather than faking attentiveness.

Good listening takes energy and discipline. If you are a good listener to yourself, you will be a good listener to others. When you respond to someone who's in need of being understood, keep the focus on the other person rather than saying, "I know how you feel. A similar thing happened to me . . ." You invalidate others' uniqueness when you compare their experiences to your own. Instead, say things that will result in the speaker's telling you more, such as, "I don't understand what you mean by . . . ," or "I'm glad you . . . ." Or touch them in a way that conveys your understanding.

When the situation is reversed, you can become a more conscious communicator. When calling someone on the telephone, you can say, "Do you have a few minutes? I really need to talk," rather than barging in with your problem.

Think about a recent conversation with a significant person in your life. Did you use the listening ladder? If not, rescript the scene incorporating the listening techniques above. How do your new actions affect the other person's responses?

A DAY IN THE LIFE

Martha   They want me to write about what happened today in group and here goes. I had an assignment to keep silent for twenty-four hours. It just about killed me and now I know why. I had to keep silent all these years! I'm two years short of fifty and this happened to me in my teens, so that's about thirty years of silence! That was why I just started screaming and *couldn't stop when I finally got to group therapy. I couldn't hold it in another minute.*

My Uncle Morty was the wealthiest of my grandmother's five sons. My father probably owed him money. That would explain a lot of things. I had an older cousin, Marguerite. She's dead now. She once warned me, "Watch out for Uncle Morty. Don't let him catch you anywhere alone, and don't go off with him alone." I had forgotten all about her warning until right now. But her warning made me very shy around Uncle Morty and that seemed to make him all the more interested in me. He had the biggest and nicest house so we always went there for the holidays. It couldn't be avoided, although come to think of it, I was sick a lot around the holidays then.

I must have been around thirteen or so; I started to blossom and his interest in me blossomed. I was a blooming young thing with rosy cheeks, pretty now when I look back, and he liked to pinch me when I went by, right in front of everybody. It was just teasing. The others would laugh. Ha ha, watch out, Uncle Morty's gonna get you! That son of a bitch! In front of the whole damn family!

I had to respect my relatives. If he said, "Marty, go to the basement and bring up a couple bottles of apple cider," I had to go. Then, with my heart racing and me breathing so hard I was wheezing, I would look for the apple cider, scared to death. It wouldn't be there, and then Uncle Morty would grab me from out of nowhere and he would kiss me and do other things to me that made me feel awful, humiliated, and I was never to tell anyone or I would get myself "into a whole lot of trouble." I would run upstairs and head for a bathroom and cry and cry. And nobody ever noticed. And I just kept silent. I want to kill that fucker! I want to mutilate him! And I always bought candy with the money I got on those holidays, fancy boxes of chocolates. And I'd eat *them all until they were gone. I never said anything, I just ate!*

•

DAY FOURTEEN

Step Study: Step Three

"Made a decision to turn our will and our lives over to the care of God as we understood Him."

The first step requires that we acknowledge our powerlessness. The second step requires that we acknowledge a power greater than ourselves. The third step requires more than just acknowledgment. It says we take action: not a small and insignificant action, but making a decision to give away the very things we value most—our will and our lives! No wonder people balk when they get to this step. Some stay on the threshold of Step Three for years and continue to struggle. That is a painful place to stay in. Others are lucky and surrender their will early, and they are grateful when they experience the Big Surprise, which simply cannot be believed or even comprehended before the step is taken. As soon as we turn our wills over to a power higher than ourselves (and that power need go no further than the power of a 12-step group), we receive more power than we were ever able to give ourselves, a great store of previously untapped resources that we can use for our own benefit and that of others.

If you are still reluctant to relinquish your will, let's examine what your self-sufficiency has done for you. Has it brought you success? Peace of mind? A rich social life? Happiness? Has it fulfilled your goals and set you free of your great craving for food? If it has, you really don't need a 12-step program, and if it hasn't, what are you really giving up?

Do we addicts even possess self-will? If we are in control of it, why are we so powerless over food? Why can't we put our wills to work for us with enthusiasm? The most enthusiastic people I know, who seem to be tapped into an infinite source of energy, bubbling up in them like a fountain of youth, are very often people who decided to turn their wills and their lives over to God.

When you are ready, Step Three will open the door. In the meantime, you can pray, "Thy will, not mine, be done." God will hear and give us the serenity we need to take that simple step that seems so impossible from outside the door and so easy once it has been opened. Take a look at the faces of people who have been in a fellowship for any length of time. Do they have the glassy-eyed look of the followers of a secret sect? Or do they seem true to themselves? There is no human being who can be trusted with our will, but we can trust a power greater than ourselves interested only in our living a life that is happy, joyous, and free. We have nothing to lose but our pain.

―――――――

ACTIVITIES FOR DAY FOURTEEN

Assignment One: Getting a Sponsor

Having come this far, you need to find a sponsor. Choose someone with long-term abstinence, someone you heard speak in meetings who inspired you, someone with whom you think you could be completely honest. You are not choosing a friend. You are choosing a bulwark of strength you will be calling every day to "turn over" your food. At the start of each day, you will telephone your sponsor and tell him or her what you plan to eat that day. In doing so, you make a mutual commitment to the program that is reestablished each day. The sponsor is also there to intervene in a slip.

You are not a burden to your sponsor. In fact, sponsors need you as much as you need them, for helping others is necessary to recovery.

Approach the person of your choice and ask him or her to be your sponsor. If that person already has too many "sponsees," he or she will help you find another. Take the telephone numbers of other people in meetings, too, and get in the habit of calling people, just to say hello. It is one of the best ways to break your isolation. The telephone is voice-activated reality. Just hearing someone from the program may be all you need to keep from giving in to a self-destructive impulse.

Assignment Two: Higher Power Questionnaire

1. How does your higher power make you feel? When did you first recognize your higher power? What were the circumstances?

2. How do you address your higher power (name)?

3. How does your higher power address you (name)?

4. Fill in the following blanks to describe your relationship with your higher power.

   My higher power is my _____

   I am my higher power's _____

5. Which statement best describes you and your higher power (check one):

   _____ I am my higher power.

   _____ I am at one with my higher power.

   _____ I am a part of my higher power.

_____ I am a child of my higher power.

_____ I am separated from my higher power.

_____ I am in conflict with my higher power.

_____ I am divorced from my higher power.

_____ I am looking for my higher power.

_____ I am a servant of my higher power.

_____ I am a house guest of my higher power.

_____ I am a tourist in my higher power's universe.

6. If you were to ask your higher power the following questions, how would your higher power answer you:

   a. Why do I have this food addiction?

   b. How can I recover from my food addiction?

   c. What is the purpose of my life?

7. If you could change your higher power in any way, what changes would you make?

8. If your higher power could change you in any way, what changes would your higher power make?

Assignment Three: Nurturing Yourself

God gives me everything I need and the strength, will, and courage to do whatever I want to do. That's the gift, but it always requires my active participation. And if God doesn't want me to have something I want, He stops me dead in my tracks. It happens every time! Sometimes it takes me a while to understand why I shouldn't have it, but I trust that it's for my good or some other higher meaning that I would never understand. I know in my heart that I want to do God's work, and God wants me to be happy, joyous, and free.

What do you want? If He wants you to have it, God will give you the gift necessary to achieve your goal.

The following visualization/meditation is designed to put you in a frame of mind to receive the kind of gift you need the most.

1. Sit comfortably, close your eyes, and relax.
2. Breathe in and out ten times and focus on your breathing.
3. In your imagination you are walking along the beach. What do you see, feel, hear, smell?
4. Now sit down on the sand. Feel the water as it comes into shore and then watch it go back out.
5. There is a gift here for you. You need to start digging in the sand until the gift appears.
6. When you have found your gift, look it over, touch it, listen to it, and smell it.
7. Place the gift in a safe place where you can enjoy it whenever you want to remember this special moment to nurture yourself.

A DAY IN THE LIFE

Chuck *I'm having a lot of difficulty with the idea of my wife coming in for family therapy. It's partially because of Gordon and his anguish over the fact that his mother is coming. From what I gather, she is a very formidable type, and a judge on top of it. Gordon has yet to really come to terms with her battering of him when he was a kid. For many a night he lay there in bed minimizing what she had done. I told him that child abuse may be more prevalent than any of us realized but that doesn't make it any more acceptable. I also told him that I thought family therapy was a great idea; they could have a safe forum where people would be fair and they could get to the bottom of things.*

The thing is, as long as it was Gordon's problem dealing with family therapy I was right there for him, supporting him all the way. But the very idea that my wife is coming here and that we could have problems shakes me badly. My wife and I have always been the solution, not the problem. My dad told me she's the best thing that ever happened to me, and warned me not to lose her. I feel shaken, like I will lose her after all, just as my dad warned. These two weeks have been the first extended period of time that I have been separated from her in thirty-five years. Why am I so shook up over her coming in here?

I know she's reacting to the fact that I'm changing. It's making her kind of suspicious, and that's the first time I've ever heard her be suspicious. I'm still processing the work we did today on the masks we made to represent the false identity we present to the world. It occurs to me that if I take my happy, smiling mask off, she's going to have to take hers off in order to feel comfortable with me. But I didn't know I was wearing one when I came in here two weeks ago, so how can she know? On the other hand, I'm not worried. I've seen too much healing going on here after family group not to have hope that it will only make what my wife and I have even better.

6

Week Three:
The Valley of Shadows

Today it's rare for patients to be hospitalized more than two or three weeks. The average length of stay for depression is nineteen days, after which patients go to a lesser level of care, such as partial hospitalization or outpatient care. Regardless, they still continue with their valuable daily journals. The diaries of Chuck, Jenny, and Martha will continue to assist you in relating to these patients as they move forward on the road to recovery.

During the past week, Chuck and Martha have had major breakthroughs. They have expressed deep, old, painful feelings that they had never released because they had never felt safe enough to do so. One of the most powerful aspects of the treatment center experience is the bonding that goes on between patients. I have found that most people become incredibly courageous, given a chance to be real, in an environment in which they feel safe. They take risks they had never dreamed of and make changes they have been yearning to make for years.

Chuck's changes are remarkable. He no longer wears his Good Guy smile. Some of the patients feel slighted because he is no longer so centered on them. Others encourage him to be whoever he feels like being. Chuck is amazed every time they accept him when he feels grumpy or noncommunicative or preoccupied. "I had no idea life could be this easy," he says. His major focus at this point is on his relationship with his wife, which can't help but change because Chuck has. However, the bond of these two self-defined "flaming codependents" is long-term and deep. There is no doubt in Chuck's mind that the two of them will work things out.

Jenny is still having trouble working on her major issues. Stories of abandonment and neglect evoke tears, but she is unable to describe what they bring up for her about her own past. She thinks she is failing in recovery, as if the whole treatment process is a test, and she is not making the grade. But she is moving forward. Because of the relationships she is developing with individuals in her group and with Bob, her primary therapist, Jenny's trust level is improving. She really wants to trust now. And she is beginning to realize that she is well liked. The patients respect her intelligence and sense of dignity, and appreciate her wry humor. They want her approval. Every now and then she can be heard laughing out loud. It is a joyful sound. Still, Jenny holds back in group situations. One time she talked about her experience at a management training retreat—a situation she described as "humiliating"—without showing any emotion, even though other people responded to her story by weeping. Jenny was moved by that response but still could not take on those feelings for herself.

With her multiple issues of sexual abuse, neglect, and battering, Martha is working hard but still has a long way to go. She has begun to make real breakthroughs in dealing with the trauma of sexual abuse and is examining it from new perspectives. Although her uncle's harassment was overt and she was not his only victim, the man's economic power in the family and position in the community protected him until his death, and this enrages Martha. Her anger spills over from the uncle onto her father's passivity. But her feelings around her father are more complicated than the blind rage she feels for her uncle's deeds. Her father did not protect her from the abuse of either her uncle or her mother. Instead, he abandoned the family until his final illness. It was Martha who took care of him during his last long hospital stay. Martha remains silent about her mother. When questions about her come up, Martha waves her hand and says, "Too much."

Martha's relationship with the other patients makes her treatment even more difficult. Although patients have been sympathetic to Martha's willingness to deal with her many issues, she has also annoyed so many individuals during the past two weeks that she feels "shunned." It's true that people definitely do not seek her out. Martha's defenses have been shaken time and again, and as a result she is more bossy and controlling than ever. Two weeks into treatment, she is at the crossroads.

Two weeks of healthy eating and abstinence from mood-altering substances are beginning to have a positive effect on your state of mind. Your mood is more even and tranquil; your highs are less high, your lows less low. You are beginning to experience real emotions, and wondering what to do about them. Week Three concentrates on expressing those emotions and then letting them go.

Two weeks of moderate daily exercise are also beginning to make you feel better about yourself. Your muscle tone is improving, more oxygen is reaching your cells, flushing out toxins and clarifying your thinking. The muscles in your legs are becoming more defined and you have fewer aches and pains.

Two weeks of meditation and positive affirmations are also beginning to have a good effect, giving you enough security to examine your behavior and identify what defenses you have been using to protect yourself and the courage to discard them.

Every now and then the real you comes out of prison and has a look around. More and more that person will dare to step forth, increasingly confident that he or she won't be abused or ignored. You know when your true self is present because you feel blissfully authentic, totally in the moment, and that moment is serene even when the activities around you are in chaos. It is the state you are striving to be in all the time, so you can be truly alive. You don't have to prove anything. Facts have little to do with the state you seek. Spirituality comes out of feeling, not logic. It moves from guesswork, intuition, feelings.

DAY FIFTEEN

Unfinished Business

It's hard to look down to the bottom of a well and see what's there. People with unfinished business from their past must be brave enough to beam a strong light into the depths, acknowledge what they find, experience the pain of it, and then express that pain. It's a shame to be hurting today for something that happened to you a long time ago.

If you have spent a lifetime suffering from old and painful memories, or spend a lot of time whistling in the dark to mask the sound of monsters rustling behind closet doors you won't open, you must get out of the poisonous environment you're in. Until you take a good look at what happened and truly feel it, you won't move on to a better place.

Anger, fear, grief, guilt, shame, resentment, and other painful feelings are negative energy, and that energy needs to be charged and disposed of in a safe place so you can get on with your life. If you have been carrying around feelings you have never expressed surrounding childhood abuse, it's time you got rid of them.

In group therapy unfinished business is called anger work, and it is highly structured because the experience can be frightening, and you may feel completely out of control. Ground rules are carefully laid beforehand so participants know what to expect. Here is a typical example: A person has been working hard in group for several weeks, bringing up long-submerged anger at an abusive parent. He has been told to write a letter to that parent and bring it to group. While he reads it, the feelings he suppressed as a child surface and begin to overwhelm him. He is ready to re-create the painful memory and express the rage and grief he has never felt safe enough to experience.

The therapist puts an empty chair in front of him, a substantial chair that will quite literally take a beating, and the patient is given a pillow. There is only one rule: He must not hurt himself or others when he expresses his anger. For instance, he can beat the pillow with an open hand, but not with a closed fist because that might hurt his hand and he has been hurt enough. He can hold the pillow in his fists and beat the chair. He can cry and rage and beat out his anger until it is gone. Sometimes more memories come up in the process of expressing anger, more pain and grief, and they, too, are acknowledged and expressed. The others in the group are there for him completely. They comfort him and validate his experience. They tell him how they have drawn strength from his courage. They hold him afterward and allow him to fully express his grief.

The power of the energy of anger is awesome, particularly in those who have never allowed themselves to tap into it. After the event, people often sleep. They wake feeling purged, as if they had lost weight, for they have. They have lost the heavy burden of unexpressed emotions they have carried all their lives. They now are free to travel light, minus the burden of the past. Taking care of unfinished business often results in permanent change: once you take your trash to the dump, you don't have a yen to go back for it afterward. The same is true for these toxic feelings: when they're gone, they're gone.

Neglect and Loss

Unfinished business is not limited to people with issues of childhood abuse. People who suffered from neglect as children often have a much more difficult time getting in touch with anger. The abuse victim has some traumatic memory to find, but victims of neglect have only a vague and amorphous nothingness. They can't point to any scars. The abuse victim has flashbacks or self-mutilates, or has memories of being hit or verbally assaulted. Victims of neglect have no picture of what they missed and no sense of what they need. If they've done without, they have no reason to think they're worthy. Neglect is the climate they've lived in, and its all-pervasive and undramatic nature is difficult to focus on.

Survivors of neglect often say, "My greatest fear is I *have* no problems." When they seek their inner child, they often find it hiding, or can't find it at all. "I ran away from home once when I was little," a victim of neglect once told me, "and when I came back, I found no one even knew I was gone." The neglect victim is often the slowest to bring up anger and grief that needs to be expressed in order to feel again. In group they are reluctant to have attention focused on themselves because their problems are so "insignificant, no big deal." "Other people have real problems," they will tell you, "I'm just neurotic."

The same difficulty is true for those who suffered religious abuse as children. It's a lot less threatening for people to bring up an abusive parent than an angry, jealous deity who has the power to read their thoughts and strike them dead! You can run away from an abusive parent, but how do you escape from an all-powerful God who can punish you for eternity?

The combined authority of parents and clergy may be too threatening to challenge, even in a safe therapeutic environment, and may be buried so deep that all that can be seen are the symptoms: human beings who cannot enjoy the simple pleasures of life, the right to live free of guilt, and to experience their own sexuality. People who suffer from religious abuse need to put that punishing "God" in the chair and go at *him* with a pillow. Afterward they find they have room for a loving God, who will help them learn to be happy, joyous, and free, as we were put on this earth to be.

Sometimes unfinished business is not so traumatic. It might be a recent or a past ungrieved-for loss. I have seen people in treatment weep for lost pets from their childhood and have been moved to tears at their outpouring of grief. It doesn't matter what the cause of the unfinished business is as much as that it has never been acknowledged, experienced, or expressed. Your reaction to reading this will confirm for you the kind of unfinished business you may have to take care of. You may have little or no reaction to it, but if you are agitated and full of negative feelings right now, my bet is you've got some bottled-up righteous anger in you that needs to be uncorked. If you want to recover, you must take care of your unfinished business. Make it your number one priority, for you deserve to live fully. Seek help.

═══════════

ACTIVITIES FOR DAY FIFTEEN

Assignment One: Unfinished Business

If you are in group therapy and feel you are ready to deal with your unfinished business, discuss it with your therapist. You may want to write a letter to the person or persons whom you have never confronted about hurtful events that occurred in your childhood that are still making you unhappy today. You may never need to confront them. The anger work is for yourself, so you can feel better. It will set you free from the prison of your past.

Assignment Two: Unfinished Business

For this exercise you will need two large sheets of drawing or wrapping paper and some colored crayons or felt-tipped markers. You might want to play some quiet, soothing background music. Before doing the exercise, take the time to close your eyes, relax your body, do some deep breathing and quiet your thoughts with meditation.

Now, take a sheet of paper and draw a picture of the happiest day of your life. Use stick figures if you like. Put in as many tangible details as you can remember—what you were wearing, what the weather was like, who was there, etc. Write a caption describing how you felt that day.

Take the second sheet of paper and draw a picture of the saddest day of your life. Again, include as many details as you can remember. Write a caption for the picture describing your feelings.

This exercise may bring up unfinished business. If it does, you need to express these deep feelings of sadness and loss to another person you can trust. Until these feelings are shared with another person, you cannot discharge their negative energy.

Assignment Three: Symptoms of Religious Abuse/Addiction

Read through the following points, taken from Father Leo Booth's book, *When God Becomes a Drug: Break-*

ing the Chains of Religious Addiction and Abuse, and check off those that evoke an emotional response.

1. Inability to think, or question information or authority
2. Black-and-white, simplistic thinking
3. Shame-based belief that you aren't good enough, or you aren't "doing it right"
4. Magical thinking that God will fix you
5. Scrupulosity: rigid, obsessive adherence to rules, codes of ethics, or guidelines
6. Uncompromising, judgmental attitudes
7. Compulsive praying, going to church or crusades, quoting scripture
8. Unrealistic financial contributions
9. Believing that sex is dirty—that our bodies and physical pleasures are evil
10. Compulsive overeating or excessive fasting
11. Conflict with science, medicine, and education
12. Progressive detachment from the real world, isolation, breakdown of relationships
13. Psychosomatic illness: sleeplessness, back pains, headaches, hypertension
14. Manipulating scripture or texts, feeling chosen, claiming to receive special messages from God
15. Trancelike state or religious high, wearing a glazed happy face
16. Cries for help; mental, emotional, physical breakdown; hospitalization

If you identify strongly with most of these symptoms you may want to explore further the impact your religious upbringing has had on your life today. Remember, true spirituality leaves people feeling happy, joyous and free.

Assignment Four: Releasing Feelings

Our minds can play tricks and "lie" to us when we're scared and unsure. Within the body old feelings are stored, yearning for release. These trapped feelings keep you tense, or tired, or always on edge. You can create a safe and loving environment in which the fear around those feelings is dissolved so that your body can be relaxed and the feelings can be released at last:

Lie on the floor. Close your eyes. Be conscious of your body. Without straining, stretch every part from your feet to your head: toes, feet, ankles, calves, knees, thighs, hips, stomach, chest, arms, hands, fingers, neck, head. Feel your whole body. Feel it vibrating with energy. Tense yourself all at once and experience your entire body's functioning; imagine all that is going on underneath your skin. Experience the wonder of that. Relax your body. Take a few deep breaths, expanding your diaphragm from the belly. Open your eyes.

You are now ready to ask yourself some questions as you lie peacefully. Notice how you are breathing, without changing that pattern. Trust that after all these years your body knows how to breathe. Notice as you breathe naturally:

—what parts of your body move when you breathe
—in what order they move
—if you are breathing through your mouth or through your nose
—if you are inhaling all the way, or if there is some restriction that prevents you from taking in a full breath
—if you empty your lungs completely when you exhale

Follow your breath and use it as a means to get to know the inner areas of your body.

Assignment Five: You are a Celebration of Life!

Every day, try to take a few minutes just to relax and be good to yourself. Close your eyes and repeat the following affirmation. Step back from your hectic life and your troubling thoughts and remember the strength within you.

Affirmation for a Troubled Mind

I know the quality of what I have
and it cannot be devalued
I know the source of all my strength
and have tapped into its power
I know the beauty of my soul
and that it can't be altered
I know I am God's child
I know I am God's child.

I know I am a treasure and my preciousness is real
I know these feelings in me now are only
  passing through
I know that it's my right to be joyous and be free
And I know I am God's child
I know I am God's child.

I feel the power of a love that is constant and all-
  giving
I feel the pull to goodness within me even now
I feel your strength embrace me as I tremble in
  this time
I can comfort my own child
I can comfort my own child.

A DAY IN THE LIFE

Jenny *It was commencement this morning. So beautiful. Roberta came here so skinny she had to sit on a pillow because her bones hurt her. Now she has color in her face and she's actually eating instead of stirring her food around. Most of all, she says this place saved her life. I remember the first time I saw her. I really saw through her, like she was barely there occu-*

pying space in front of me. It was like her spirit was
leaving her, and I could sense death around her. And I
watched her get better. Once in a psychodrama, doing
an activity called "Kiss the Baby," she played the role
of someone who told the person playing the baby,
"Come on, give us a kiss," and Martha had her first
breakthrough. This woman Roberta just radiated. I
stood next to her and felt it. She felt so good being able
to help this person who is so difficult to love.

So anyway, I'm glad to be here today, and I told
Roberta "Godspeed" when I kissed her goodbye. That's
what my grandmother always says. And I know I'm
supposed to write about ME ME ME and my FEEL-
INGS FEELINGS FEELINGS but at least I can feel
things for others. At least I'm not numb anymore. And
I have a real friendship with a man. At first I felt the
old pitter-patter because Gordon fits into the unavailable mode. I mean, this man has got it out for his mother
and what she did to him. He would not be a terrifically
nurturing guy to fall in love with. But now I know
Gordon, not as a stand-in for the main man in my life
so far—my dad—but for himself. He confides in me and
I in him. He trusts me and I trust him. I feel so comfortably close around him, like when I was a little kid with
my dad.

Another glad thing: my roommate Peggy. Although
I could never be as abrupt as she is, like when she tells
Martha, "Lady, don't flap your mouth at me," she
makes me think about how I could communicate how
I really feel when people cross my boundaries, in a style
that I'm comfortable with. Let me see. I'll practice here:
When you give me unasked-for advice, Martha, I feel
irritated. Angry? Invaded? Intimidated? Less than you?
All of the above. I need . . . Let me see now . . . I need
. . . Isn't that strange? I just draw a complete blank on
what I need. Better take that to group tomorrow.

•

DAY SIXTEEN

Unfinished Business: Trauma

A trauma is a catastrophic event that changes the way you perceive the world and the way you view your place in it. In children this perception becomes frozen in the moment of trauma and remains that way unless treated. Untreated, the effects of trauma are expressed in the adult as obsessive thinking; unexplained terror; perfectionism; hypercritical, controlling, rigid, and compulsive behavior; and a shame-based identity.

In most survivors of trauma there is no memory of the actual event, or even of entire years surrounding it. Commonly they have gaps in their life history that cannot be accounted for. Although the trauma may be well hidden, the results are obvious to one and all. As adults, the survivors of trauma become hopeless, feel helpless and stuck in their defenses, and turn to addictions to relieve or numb their pain.

The causes of trauma are multiple: the sudden death of a parent, war or natural disaster, witnessing a crime, battering, especially by the significant parent, and sexual abuse. We live in a violent world, and many of us are victims. While we may never be clear as to exactly what happened, we can change the way we have learned to adapt. First of all, we need to acknowledge our past adaptability, and the fact that by defending ourselves, we did after all find a way to survive. But we also need to acknowledge our right to happiness. Survival is not enough. We want to be happy, joyous, and free. We want to thrive! Reliance on defenses, no matter how effective, may result in feeling safe but never result in feeling free.

ACTIVITIES FOR DAY SIXTEEN

Looking for Safety

If you are going to live your life looking for safety, you are going to have a dreary life, and maybe not even a safe one. In this life there is no guarantee. Even if you are physically safe, you may not know emotional safety. I try to create a safe place for traumatized people at my treatment centers because I know how important it is for me to feel safe. We provide a group of loving, caring professionals whose goal is to get patients to the point where they feel safe enough to unload their burden of depression and reveal what's really eating them. You need to do that for yourself at home.

Assignment One: What Makes Me Feel Safe—People

Make a list of the people around whom you feel safe, past and present.

Assignment Two: What Makes Me Feel Safe—Places

Make another list of places, past and present, where you feel safe—free to be yourself minus the fear that brings on the mask and the arsenal of defenses.

Assignment Three: What Makes Me Feel Safe—Things

Make a third list of the material things you need to feel safe: a paid-up mortgage, a savings account, a lot of insurance—whatever it is.

Assignment Four: Assessment

Look over your three lists and make an observation about your patterns: What is repeated? What has changed? What does feeling safe really mean to you?

Assignment Five: Rewriting the Fairy Tale

One of the aspects of childhood that remains frozen by early trauma is a childish perception of the world, namely, a belief in magic. In the adult, that belief often becomes increasingly fervent and fantasies veil reality. I have met some women who, years later, are still waiting for their prince to come, clinging to the fantasy and always looking for the magic, the quick and easy fix.

Staying in the magic mode keeps a person stuck, usually being "very good" while waiting for something to happen. Taking that first step in giving up your fantasies is a giant step, and there will be great resistance. The following activity is a tool for letting go of your delusions and taking control of your life. You'll learn that the only magic solutions to life's problems are solutions that you actively initiate.

Choose the fairy tale you most strongly identify with and give it a new ending, one which shows you acting in your own best interests and being true to your integrity. Is there a moral to your fairy tale? What is that moral? What qualities do you have that could be put to good use to enable you to enact the new ending to your fairy tale? An example may be *Cinderella*. Instead of staying home waiting for her prince to come, the story may end with Cinderella leaving her cruel home and seeking her fortune, using her courage and wit to find her own happiness.

Assignment Three: Reassociating

"Dissociation" is the term used for the disconnection from the spirit that is the result of trauma. This visualization is a tool for reassociating what has been disconnected. It will also help you visualize your inner child not as a victim, but as a being with great beauty and power, one who has a great zest for feeling, loving, seeing, creating.

Lie down comfortably and close your eyes. Search your imagination for the child you were, and when it is clear in your mind, ask that child, "Do you want to play with me?" Look at its little face light up with happiness. Let your child lead you wherever it is safe to have fun—to the playground, a back yard, the beach. And together play in the sand, climb hills, do cartwheels across the lawn. Envision playing until your child becomes tired. Then take it in your arms and rock your child gently until it falls asleep.

A DAY IN THE LIFE

Martha *I just found out my brother is going to come. He is actually going to leave the store in the care of my sister-in-law Susan and spend the time with me. Can you believe it? I've hardly spoken to him in three years, since the big blowup. I'm petrified of him. He's like mother, such a sharp tongue. Every time I think about him coming, I get sick to my stomach.*

•

DAY SEVENTEEN

Childhood Sexual Abuse

I define sexual abuse as any behavior that causes people to feel fear, shame, and a sense that something is wrong with them. Its prevalence among children is society's "dirty little secret." Nationwide, studies indicate that around 16–17 percent of the population have been sexually abused as children. Studies conducted on people with eating disorders reveal a much higher percentage than in the general population. In a survey of five hundred people who have gone through my treatment program, 27 percent said they were incest survivors. A study by Father Leo Booth documents the same percentage among nuns. In the broader category of sexual abuse (including acts committed by people outside the family) the statistics are truly shocking. In one survey of patients with eating disorders, 64 percent said they had undergone coercive sexual events as children. Seventy-five percent was the statistic given on the television special on the subject of eating disorders called *Kate's Secret,* starring Meredith Baxter, and I have read other studies that claim a figure among the addict population as high as 80 percent.

There is a logical reason for the high incidence of sexual abuse among people with eating disorders. Food is usually the only mood-altering substance available to children, and they turn to it for solace to numb their feelings of rage and shame. Many develop a lifelong emotionally charged relationship with food that eventually leads to an eating disorder. Among people with eating disorders, the incidence of sexual abuse is the highest among bulimics. It is, after all, a disease of secrecy.

One of the most damaging aspects of childhood abuse is this element of secrecy. Bruno Bettelheim made the observation that when the pattern of abuse among children is societal—the unfortunate "norm"—they do not take on the guilt of their oppressors. Children abused out in the open, particularly when it is a fate they see shared by others, suffer far less psychological damage than children who were abused in private. Secrecy distorts reality and makes the child take on the blame and the shame the oppressor should be feeling. These feelings are then turned inward on themselves because they have nowhere else to go, and fear of discovery keeps the feelings buried, because the abused children were frequently threatened into remaining silent or convinced what happened was their fault.

In order to escape from an intolerable situation, the sexually abused develop dissociating mechanisms, taking leave of their bodies to live in their heads. Some take leave of reality itself and develop multiple personalities. Others simply learn to "go away," to leave their bodies mentally and emotionally. The ultimate abandonment is the forced exile from the self, and it is the tragic legacy of childhood sexual abuse.

Although all forms of sexual abuse are abhorrent, incest is the most damaging because it occurs within the family circle where children are supposed to be safe from harm. In the case of incest by a parent, the event may be so traumatic it is completely repressed, or children may create a self-protective myth out of the incident that *they* are responsible for the behavior of the parent. Because they cannot survive knowing the parent they depend on for nurturance is also abusing them, they take on the parent's guilt and minimize what happened, or repress it entirely, often disconnecting from their bodies in the process. Many never get reconnected. One of my patients with a long history of deep depression had been to six treatment centers before coming to "Your Life Matters." At none of them had the issue of incest ever been addressed, let alone pursued. When she felt safe enough at the center, she let herself remember, and her lifelong depression has since lifted. She came back from exile and is living in her body again, able to feel both pleasant and hurtful emotions. Getting reconnected doesn't mean the end of feeling bad, just the beginning of feeling anything.

It is amazing to me how many of my sexually abused patients come from very religious homes. The incidence of incest is unusually high among the highly religious, as if the unnatural damming up of the sexual urge common among them causes desperate people to seek other outlets. All too often the outlet of least resistance is a child. Sexually abused children must learn to live somehow with contradictory moral messages. They are often taught that sex is bad, and that they should watch out for strangers. Yet a relative does the bad thing to them, often the same person who said it was wrong. In an attempt to make sense of the hypocrisy, children create explanations for themselves in which reality becomes badly fractured.

Traditionally, rape victims were blamed for their victimization, and the same holds true for children who are sexually molested. They must have "asked for it," especially if they were desperate for affection and attention. I know one five-year-old girl who begged to go to confession to relieve herself of her guilt after being sexually abused by an older brother. Survivors of sexual abuse must be told again and again that they are not responsible for what was done to them.

When sexually abused children grow up, they continue to live in a state of altered reality, using food or drugs to dull the troublesome feelings they can't control or comprehend and that won't go away. If you were sexually abused as a child and have not dealt with the issue, you need help. If you are wondering whether you have repressed memories of sexual abuse, believe me, no one makes up such an unhappy past for him- or herself. The seeds can be planted in someone's mind, but they will not germinate if the event didn't take place. If you have a secret you're keeping from yourself, your autonomic nervous system will respond to the memory prodding and begin to work on bringing up all the repressed emotions that must be dealt with.

You cannot deal with this issue alone. There is a profile of a survivor of childhood sexual abuse in today's workbook section. If your identification with it is high, I strongly recommend you go into therapy. If you can't, there are sexual abuse hotlines and 12-step Incest

Survivor and Adult Children of Alcoholics groups all over the country. Contact one in your area.

ACTIVITIES FOR DAY SEVENTEEN

Assignment One: How the Story Changed

The past only matters in how it's affecting you today. Today you are going to write a story that will help you clarify that connection. It is a short story, consisting of three paragraphs. The first paragraph begins "Once upon a time," and it tells how someone, yourself or a fictional character, or even an animal, protected him- or herself in the past. The second paragraph begins "When he/she grew up" and tells how that person continued the behavior learned in the past. The third paragraph begins "The story changed when" and tells how that person learned different patterns of behavior to cope with life. It will reveal how you would feel about yourself with a new style of interacting compared to the old style that didn't work, and it will begin motivating you to put that new style into practice.

Assignment Two: Profile of a Survivor of Childhood Sexual Abuse

Check off the characteristics that are true for you:

1. _____ You have no memory of childhood, or only brief flashes, such as being held on someone's lap.
2. _____ You feel guilty a lot for no reason.
3. _____ You have a history of inability to sustain a love relationship.
4. _____ You frequently indulge in short pursuit-

and-revenge love affairs, earning a reputation for being a Jezebel or a "lady killer."

5. _____ You consistently find the excitement of a triangular love affair (for instance, involvement with someone who is married) more exciting than involvement without the need for secrecy.

6. _____ You experience flashbacks in a waking state: brief, vivid, and disturbing images of a sexual nature that provoke strong anxiety.

7. _____ You have recurring dreams of a sexual nature, often involving body parts or unidentified people, that provoke strong anxiety.

8. _____ You have difficulty establishing boundaries, either letting everyone in or keeping everyone out.

9. _____ You practice all-or-nothing extremes in sexual behavior such as celibacy or promiscuity.

10. _____ You are often strongly drawn to people who abuse you.

11. _____ You are obsessed with love relationships and only feel alive when seeking or receiving affection.

12. _____ You feel disconnected from your body, as if it were numb from the neck down.

13. _____ In order to achieve orgasm, you often fantasize scenes of bondage in which you are coerced into the sexual act.

14. _____ You have an excessive need to please.

15. _____ You practice self-mutilation, scratching or cutting yourself until you bleed, either consciously or in your sleep.

16. _____ You have a problem with moral ambivalence and often seek the opinion of others about a moral issue because you don't trust your own.

17. _____ You are overly protective of others.

18. _____ You are manipulative rather than assertive in dealing with others.

19. _____ You fear the consequences of change.

20. _____ You are uncomfortable when good things happen to you and become anxious if good feelings are prolonged.

21. _____ When you were young, you felt older than your peers and never really felt like a child.

22. _____ You have magical expectations of other people and the world.

23. _____ You have abnormally high expectations of yourself that you can't possibly meet.

24. _____ You have a pattern of failure in meeting and satisfying your own needs.

25. _____ You expect people to read your mind. (Please guess my awful secret.)

26. _____ As a child you felt special and believed you were the favorite.

27. _____ You have a tendency to "space out."

28. _____ You are secretive and have trouble trusting others.

29. _____ You generally feel inauthentic, or as if you wear a mask.

30. _____ You have a great desire to dance but are inhibited and can't let go.

31. _____ You have a strong identification with the oppressed and are active in human rights or animal rights causes.

If you checked more than twenty of the characteristics, you need to consider finding someone to help you. Not thinking you are worthy of giving yourself something you really need is part of the profile. (See Day Twenty-six, Choosing a Therapist.)

Assignment Three: Mirror Affirmation

This is a powerful affirmation, and it will assist you in bringing up repressed memories. If you fit the above profile of a survivor of childhood sexual abuse, do not use it unless you are getting some kind of therapeutic help.

Look directly into your eyes and repeat this affirmation three times, in the morning and again at night before you go to bed:

> [Call yourself by name], you are wonderful and
> I love you.
> This is one of the best days of your life.
> Everything is working for your greatest good.
> Whatever you need to know is revealed to you.
> Whatever you need will come to you.
> All is well.

A DAY IN THE LIFE

Chuck I'm looking at my lifelong addictive patterns and I'm seeing how connected they are to loneliness. I spent my early years on a farm where there were no kids my age, so food became my friend. It was waiting for me when I came home from school each day. I remember my dad telling me when I was in kindergarten that if I didn't stop eating so much I'd end up looking like a washing machine, but I've got photographs of me at that age, and I look like a relatively normal little boy. Nevertheless, I did it. By the age of twelve I was huge, just like my dad said I would be.

I was transferred into a school system where I was an outsider, and I was the brunt of everyone's fat jokes. My classmates got a big kick out of watching me run in gym. To this day I can feel the humiliation I experienced when I watched a boy do an imitation of me. I remained an outsider for many years. I didn't fit in, so I ate.

The loneliness and isolation I felt so much those growing-up years made me determined never to be lonely again. The greatest luck of my life was meeting Jean. We hit it off from the first date. We wanted to have more children, but Jean's health couldn't take it. But all the years we raised children, there were always one or two extra plates at the table because kids gravitated to us, kids in trouble, or just in need of being in a happy home for a while. We did provide that, a happy home, but boy, did the two of us pay a price for it. We're exhausted, depleted, and we don't know quite what to do with ourselves.

Now that I've discovered the pattern of my addiction, I see the damage it has done and its tremendous power. I see how my number-one obligation to myself is to keep from being in its thrall, not for the rest of my life, but for now and the next few hours, one day at a time. I can handle that.

·

DAY EIGHTEEN

Sexual Dysfunction

When people grow up in dysfunctional homes, rarely is their adult sexuality healthy. It has been thwarted along with all their other interpersonal responses. The ability to enjoy sexuality is a clear indicator of a healthy mentality and should be everyone's goal. We are all entitled to enjoy our God-given sexuality without fear or guilt.

Some causes of sexual inadequacy are easy to resolve, such as sexual ignorance, in which case education alone can change a person's values, attitudes, and beliefs. Failure to communicate desires is another problem that can easily be resolved, although many people need to overcome their belief that they don't have a right to experience full sexual pleasure before they can be specific about what they want from their partners. Discord in a relationship can also be the cause of sexual dysfunction, in which case the sexual life of a couple will be adversely affected until they can work out the real problem. Other people use sexuality as a power play, because they feel they have to be in control. They need to learn how to disengage from the power struggle by exploring why they feel they must be in control, and what would happen if they surrendered to the other person. Merely recognizing that a power play is going on becomes part of the solution.

Other causes, such as early sexual trauma, are much more difficult to resolve. When children experience a traumatic violation of their boundaries, they have a tremendously difficult time trusting others when they grow up. They are afraid of intimacy and are confused about what it means to get close to someone. They need to learn that intimacy is about shared experiences in the here and now, and that can sometimes but not necessarily include sex.

They also have a lot of trouble enjoying the sexual act. It's hard for them to "be there." If they have repressed their memories of childhood sexual abuse, they must disconnect from what is happening in the present to keep from remembering what happened in the past. Others can give but not experience pleasure in order to maintain their sense of goodness. Whereas some survivors are frigid, letting no one in, others become promiscuous, letting everyone in. Many prostitutes were sexually abused as children.

Sometimes people with a history of childhood sexual abuse indulge in sadomasochistic rituals because they feel a need to be punished for past sins before pleasure can be experienced, or they create bondage fantasies while having sex. Pretending they are being coerced into the act eliminates the conflict they are having over wanting to experience sexual pleasure. Other people who have been sexually abused describe how they jump into threatening and dangerous situations instead of experiencing small pleasures with a "safe" person.

It is also common for these victims of early sexual trauma to sabotage pleasure in other areas of their life. If a job situation or a relationship is going well, something must be wrong. Their fractured sense of reality tells them that if they are experiencing pleasure, there must be some kind of sin involved, and for that they must be punished. Often they prefer to self-punish because that way they have some control over how and when it happens, as well as its severity. Self-mutilation is another way they experience a false sense of control over their impulses to self-punish, as well as a way they attempt to reduce anger.

Like food, alcohol, work, or any other source of pleasure, sex can be abused to the point of addiction. It follows the same pattern of progressive self-destructiveness of other addictions, only it masquerades as love. But the sex addict is not really looking for a satisfying relationship. Although that may seem to be the goal, addictive sex objectifies the partner, which makes love and mutual caring an impossibility. The kind of isolation the sex addict feels is perhaps the loneliest of all, because the ritual that brings two people the closest together is for the sex addict a solitary act. Even then he or she is alone, more isolated than ever.

In the early stages of sexual addiction, people use their sexuality to express not love but power, frustration, or anger, or as a form of relief from tension or loneliness. Women will have sex when they don't desire it rather than risk losing a relationship, or out of a feeling of obligation. Later on, use escalates to abuse, then progresses to obsession to the point where sex addicts become powerless to control their behavior. In their desperate search for tenderness, they become addicted to the excitement of sexual conquest instead, perpetually on the roam for the next partner.

Sexual addiction takes many forms. For some it becomes complete abstinence, a form of sexual anorexia, or is limited to masturbation. For others it has a binge-and-starve quality: periods of intense activity followed by periods of no activity at all and an overall feeling of numbness. No matter what form it takes, the common denominator is loneliness. Whether acting out or not, the emptiness remains, and the relief experienced has little to do with true bonding.

There are three kinds of 12-step programs for sex addicts, with differing beliefs and aims. The goal of Sex Addicts Anonymous is sexual health and a desire to stop compulsive sexual behavior. Its definition of sobriety does not include abstinence from the sexual act but from "the compulsive, destructive behaviors that rendered our lives unmanageable." Sex and Love Addicts Anonymous deals primarily with self-respect, and its requirement for membership is a desire to stop living out a pattern of sex and love addiction, which it defines as "any sexual or emotional act which, once engaged in, leads to loss of control over rate, frequency or duration of its recurrence, resulting in worsening self-destructive consequences."

Sexaholics Anonymous believes in sexual sobriety and identifies sexual addiction as lust. Its concept of sobriety is the most limiting of the three groups, disallowing any form of sex with oneself or with someone other than a spouse, meaning single people do not indulge in sexual activity.

If you feel a need to belong to a group that addresses problems of addictive sex and love, these groups may be helpful. I find their meetings dignified, and they do not discuss problems in an explicit or offensive way. They are also careful about screening newcomers.

ACTIVITIES FOR DAY EIGHTEEN

Assignment One: Sexual Values, Fears, and Prejudices

Complete the following sentences:

1. The way I learned about sex was . . .
2. My most awkward experience with sexuality in adolescence was . . .
3. Watching my parents, I learned . . .
4. My church taught me . . .
5. One of the unspoken messages I got from my mother about me was . . .
6. One of the unspoken messages I got from my father about myself was . . .
7. When I contemplate my mother's impact on my sexual development . . .
8. When I contemplate my father's impact on my sexual development . . .
9. _____ gave me a positive sense of my sexuality.
10. I knew I was a boy/girl when . . .
11. In my family the good thing about being a boy/girl was . . .
12. My first sexual memories are . . .
13. If it turns out I don't need my parents' permission to be a man/woman . . .
14. If it turns out I don't need my parents' permission to be a sexual being . . .
15. If I were fully willing to own and experience my sexuality . . .

16. The most sensual thing is . . .
17. The sexiest thing about me is . . .
18. I like sex when . . .
19. I'm good at sex when . . .

What have you learned about your sexuality from completing these sentences?

Assignment Two: Questionnaire: Are You a Sex and Love Addict?

(Taken from a pamphlet developed by The Augustine Fellowship—Sex and Love Addicts Anonymous)

Yes   No

____ ____ 1. Have you ever tried to control how much sex to have or how often you would see someone?

____ ____ 2. Do you find yourself unable to stop seeing a specific person even though you know that seeing this person is destructive to you?

____ ____ 3. Do you feel that you don't want anyone to know about your sexual or romantic activities?
Do you feel you need to hide these activities from others—friends, family, co-workers, counselors, etc.?

____ ____ 4. Do you get "high" from sex and/or romance?
Do you crash?

____ ____ 5. Have you had sex at inappropriate times, in inappropriate places, and/or with inappropriate people?

_____ _____ 6. Do you make promises to yourself or rules for yourself concerning your sexual or romantic behavior that you find you cannot follow?

_____ _____ 7. Have you had or do you have sex with someone you don't/didn't want to have sex with?

_____ _____ 8. Do you believe that sex and/or a relationship will make your life bearable?

_____ _____ 9. Have you ever felt that you HAD to have sex?

_____ _____ 10. Do you believe that someone can "fix" you?

_____ _____ 11. Do you keep a list, written or otherwise, of the number of partners you've had?

_____ _____ 12. Do you feel desperation or uneasiness when you are away from your lover or sexual partner?

_____ _____ 13. Have you lost count of the number of sexual partners you've had?

_____ _____ 14. Have you or do you have sex regardless of the consequences (e.g., the threat of being caught, the risk of contracting herpes, gonorrhea, AIDS, etc.)?

_____ _____ 15. Do you find that you have a pattern of repeating bad relationships?

_____ _____ 16. Do you feel that your only (or major) value in a relationship is your ability to perform sexually, or provide an emotional fix?

_____ _____ 17. Do you feel like a lifeless puppet unless there is someone around with whom you can flirt? Do you feel that you're not "really alive" unless you are with your sexual/romantic partner?

—— —— 18. Do you feel entitled to sex?

—— —— 19. Do you find yourself in a relationship that you cannot leave?

—— —— 20. Have you ever threatened your financial stability or standing in the community by pursuing a sexual partner?

—— —— 21. Do you believe that the problems in your "love life" result from not having enough of or the right kind of sex, or from continuing to remain with the "wrong" kind of person?

—— —— 22. Have you ever had a serious relationship threatened or destroyed because of your outside sexual activity?

—— —— 23. Do you feel that life would have no meaning without a love relationship or without sex? Do you feel that you would have no identity if you were not someone's lover?

—— —— 24. Do you find yourself flirting or sexualizing with someone even if you do not mean to?

—— —— 25. Does your sexual and/or romantic behavior affect your behavior?

—— —— 26. Do you have sex and/or "relationships" to try to deal with or escape from life's problems?

—— —— 27. Do you feel uncomfortable about your masturbation because of the frequency with which you masturbate, the fantasies you engage in, the props you use, and/or the places in which you do it?

_____ _____ 28. Do you engage in the practices of voyeurism, exhibitionism, etc., in ways that bring you discomfort and pain?

_____ _____ 29. Do you find yourself needing greater and greater variety and energy in your sexual or romantic activities just to achieve an "acceptable" level of physical and emotional relief?

_____ _____ 30. Do you need to have sex or "fall in love" to feel like a "real man" or "real woman"?

_____ _____ 31. Do you feel that your sexual and romantic behavior is about as rewarding as hijacking a revolving door? Are you jaded?

_____ _____ 32. Are you unable to concentrate on other areas of your life because of thoughts or feelings you are having about another person or about sex?

_____ _____ 33. Do you find yourself obsessing about a specific person or sexual act even though these thoughts bring pain, craving, or discomfort?

_____ _____ 34. Have you ever wished you could stop or control your sexual and romantic activities for a given period of time? Have you ever wished you could be less emotionally dependent?

_____ _____ 35. Do you find the pain in your life increasing no matter what you do? Are you afraid that deep down you are unacceptable?

—— —— 36. Do you feel that you lack dignity and wholeness?

—— —— 37. Do you feel that your sexual and/or romantic life affects your spiritual life in a negative way?

—— —— 38. Do you feel that your life is unmanageable because of your sexual/romantic behavior or your excessive dependency needs?

—— —— 39. Have you ever thought that there might be more you could do with your life if you were not so driven by sexual and romantic pursuits?

If you have answered "yes" to more than half of the forty questions, you may be using sex as a way to seek relief rather than as an expression of love. You may find it helpful to attend a Sex and Love Addicts meeting. (Call your local Alcoholics Anonymous switchboard, or call 1-800-362-2644 for the Sexual Addiction Access Helpline.)

Assignment Three: Sexual Dysfunction Checklists

According to Masters and Johnson, sexual dysfunction is a "condition in which physical responses of sexual function are impaired." The impairment is often caused by the food addict's negative body image and frozen feelings. The following checklists will help you decide whether you have a sexual dysfunction. Put a check mark next to all symptoms you identify with.

Symptoms of Sexual Dysfunction

—— 1. Impotency, or the inability for a male to have or maintain an erection with a partner.

_____ 2. Premature ejaculation, or the difficulty for a man to delay orgasm for a "reasonable" amount of time.

_____ 3. Difficulty in bringing oneself to orgasm.

_____ 4. Vaginismus, or involuntary spasms by the vaginal muscles that prevent penetration.

_____ 5. Frigidity, which includes the failure to reach orgasm, a lack of sexual interest, difficulty in becoming sexually aroused, withholding sexually in a relationship, unresponsiveness to a partner's lovemaking.

_____ 6. Inability or difficulty in expressing sexual needs.

_____ 7. Little or no foreplay.

_____ 8. Discomfort or out of touch with body.

_____ 9. Sex given no priority.

_____ 10. Rigid sex roles or positions/unwilling to deviate from sexual patterns.

_____ 11. Inhibition, e.g., dressing in the dark.

_____ 12. Sense of shame or repulsion about sex.

_____ 13. Performance anxiety.

Patterns of Sexual Dysfunction in Food Addicts

_____ 14. ANOREXIA. Anorexics withhold sex to avoid and numb their sexual feelings and fears. By denying their bodies food, they are able to remain childlike and prepubescent, even to the point of no longer having periods.

_____ 15. BULIMIA. Bulimics are very seductive and give out mixed messages of "Come here/go away." They usually have a history of sexually acting out.

_____ 16. COMPULSIVE OVEREATERS. They protect themselves and hide behind their weight. They often regain weight out of fear of sexually acting out, and use the weight to set sexual boundaries for themselves.

If you checked *any* of these symptoms you are experiencing diminished pleasure in this important area of life. If you checked more than five, I recommend you seek help.

Assignment Four: What Gives You Pleasure?

For each of the five senses—sight, hearing, smell, touch, and taste, complete the sentence, "I get pleasure when I . . ." For example, the colors of a sunset may turn you on, or the sound of church bells on a quiet Sunday morning. Be specific about what gives you pleasure. Don't give up if you can't answer right away. We are so accustomed to denying ourselves the ordinary, everyday pleasures!

A DAY IN THE LIFE

Jenny The tears won't stop since psychodrama, when I did the exercise about loss. Why does the death of my dog affect me so deeply? Why do I feel more grief over her loss than any other loss in my life? The strength of these feelings just amazes me. I just realized what it is about the dog that I miss so much: she was always there, waiting for me. Once I watched her through a store window as she waited for me to come out. Her eyes never moved from the door, the last place she caught sight of me. Her faithfulness and her constancy are what I need so much and didn't get anywhere else. I'm doing what Bob suggested and keeping this pen moving in my diary for three minutes without stopping and seeing what comes out. But this hurts! Where is it coming from and why won't it go away? It feels like something is taking hold of chunks of my insides and tearing me and ripping me and stomping on me and jumping on me and screaming screaming screaming I want to SCREAM so bad I want to tear out my throat with the sound. Don't you understand? I WANT to make a loud noise I want to be BAD and create a scene. I can see the look on my mother's face if I did. But I love my mother. She's wonderful. She's not like the monsters I hear about here. She's a good and hard-working person who took an extra job so we could live in a safe neighborhood, who's miserable because she's so lonely all the time. I bet she's on the freeway right now, just driving around. I know she's miserable because everybody's somewhere else. Her ex-husband, my dad, is right now sitting on the couch with his new wife and she's nice, not like a wicked stepmother. And she's always been nothing but good and generous to me and their two little kids, one who has bronchitis so he can't come to family therapy, FUCK HIM JUST FUCK HIM AND THE WHOLE FUCKING BUNCH! Let them all go to hell! Let them all get bronchitis and just cough themselves to death! Hey Bob, is that anger or what? I mean I'M REALLY MAD AT ALL OF THEM! Mr. Nice Guy, my dad. He never raised a voice, or laid a hand on me, or was anything but respectful, and I can't take up group time talking about him when there are fathers who are monsters, rapists, batterers. My God, I don't believe the things I hear. But now I'm supposed to focus on me and not write about anybody else for a while. OK: Me and Dad. He and mom broke up when I was ten. It was no big deal. No yelling, no scene or anything. My grandma was so sad, though. She loved my dad, thought Mom had chosen very well. I spent that summer at her farm in South Carolina. I rode horses and ran and ran and ran and rode and rode and rode. I've never thought about that summer until now. My grandma saved my life. No one seemed to remember

I was supposed to hurt. I didn't act hurt around her because that would have made her feel bad, but as I look back on her that summer she was there, constantly, and my grandpa, too, although he was blind and kind of crochety. See how mild and nothing my problems are? My grandfather was blind so sometimes he acted grumpy. Imagine coming up with that in group and beating up on a chair because my dad and mom got divorced. My oh my! Bob, I'm hurting so bad. Why does it have to hurt like this? Why can't I cry out loud or make a loud sound, scream and roar and rage? If I could only make the sounds MARTHA makes! I think I could get better if I could make those sounds. Will you help me? I'm so ANGRY!!!!!!

·

DAY NINETEEN

Codependency and Addictive Relationships

"Codependency" is a fairly new word, but it describes a behavior trait as old as Adam and Eve. Dysfunctional families produce codependent behavior, which is defined in many ways: Codependence is focusing one's life on another person and calling it caring. It is doing things for others they can and should do for themselves. It is slavery by mutual agreement: two needy people don't want to focus on their own problems so they obsess on each other's. It's giving away your whole pie and leaving nothing for yourself.

Here is my favorite definition of codependent people: When they die, someone else's life flashes before their eyes!

"No man is an island." Everyone in this world is dependent on other people. Codependency is a matter of degree, and usually that degree is lopsided: one person gives 80 percent and the other 20. Here's a joke illustrating codependency: There was a mouse who asked an elephant if he could make love to her. She said, "Okay." While the mouse went at it, a coconut fell on the elephant's head. "Ouch," she said, and the mouse replied, "Oh! Did I hurt you?" That's a codependent talking.

No relationship is ever fifty–fifty all the time, but if the percentages are way off center, it's codependency—one is giving far too much and the other far too little. The person who cares too much is often staying in the relationship not because of the benefits derived from it but because of fear of what would happen if he or she was faced with being alone. That fear far outweighs any pain suffered in the lopsided give-and-take of the codependent relationship.

The paradox is, in order for two people to be close, they have to be separate. The most comfortable relationship occurs when two people can live alone with each other. That's interdependency. If one needs the other too much, codependency results. If I must give up me to be loved by you, the price is too great. If I have never learned to love myself, I *can't* love you. That's the tragedy of most codependent relationships.

The subject of codependency comes up in the treatment of addiction because for many addicts it is the bottom-line obsession. I know many people who went into a 12-step program to stop drinking, only to become addicted to food. Then, when they went into recovery from that addiction, they turned to a relationship to obsess on. It's the addicts' dilemma to be constantly compelled to fill themselves up with an external element. Relationships are the most difficult addiction of all; we don't expect food, alcohol, or other substances to love us back! We experience feelings related to love, but in relationships it's give, give, give.

Addicts have a tendency to codependent relationships. They may manage to function intellectually, and even be highly esteemed in their profession and in their community. Terrified they have no real identity of their own, they often bond with people who are emotional "takers" and are grateful for the chance to obsess on someone else rather than on their own seeming insignificance. They have a tendency to think the source of the stress is work or other external factors, but the source is always internal, and comes out of relationships.

No amount of relaxation techniques, meditation, assertiveness training, or affirmations will remove the stress caused by a codependent relationship. That doesn't mean we put off practicing these things until recovery. We just have to know they are not going to take away stress. Only developing boundaries so that the flow of the relationship goes in as well as out will reduce stress to the degree of manageability.

Relationship addiction is really about someone else making you feel okay. It's needing another person to fill your cup. If you have low self-esteem and difficulty loving yourself, and if someone else is necessary to make you feel whole or alive, then you will undoubtedly suffer severe withdrawal symptoms if the loved one leaves, especially abruptly. It is then that the addiction can really be seen for what it is.

There are plenty of people caught up in relationship addictions, men and women alike. They go from one relationship to another, on emotional bender after emotional bender, to keep from having to face themselves and their terrifying inner emptiness. As someone I know pointed out, it's one thing to have a love affair with food or booze, but at least you don't expect it to call you on the phone.

I once knew an alcoholic who hid bottles all over his house, fearing that one day he would find himself without booze. That horrible day happened, on a Sunday when the liquor stores were closed. He walked for miles until, nearly crawling on his hands and knees in desperation, he found a bartender who sold him a bottle of vodka. Then, as soon as the bottle was in his possession, he was fine. He went home and didn't even take a drink. Having the alcohol in his house was more important than drinking it, and as soon as his relationship to the substance had been restored, he was all right again. That's what I see in many relationship addicts. It doesn't matter whether they're intimate with the object of their desires, they just need the body around to be okay. It's not who the person is that matters, it's just not being able to tolerate the state of being alone. If not being alone is your goal in life, you are undoubtedly a codependent, and you have most likely had a lot of difficulty establishing and sustaining relationships.

In gambling, anticipation of the game is more exciting than the actual act. It's a life-and-death situation, so the anticipation is more rewarding. The same thing happens with food: the anticipation of the act of eating it is more rewarding than the act itself. That also applies for relationships: the dreaming of what's going to happen is more rewarding than the actual relationship.

As long as other people are needed to form your identity, you will be living in an emotionally addictive state. As long as you are operating out of externals, where your identity comes from what you do or who you're with rather than who you are, you will never achieve the separateness that is necessary for two people to be truly intimate. Working on that identity is the last thing most codependents want, because they're so used to focusing on others. The thought of working on themselves fills them with despair, for it means a complete turnaround in their lifelong direction, and relinquishing the idea of waiting for someone else to provide them with a sense of self. They hate having to face the realization that it won't ever happen.

When codependents decide to break free from their addiction to a relationship and seek their own identity, the people who depend on them to stay the same will do everything possible to change their minds. They will create emergencies, threaten to leave, and act out in all sorts of diverting ways. Because they will inevitably meet this opposition, codependents need help, and I believe the best kind available for codependency issues is group therapy. Although one-on-one therapy has its place, working out problems with a group helps unmask the incredible delusions that go along with relationship addictions. Hearing stories similar to your situation rather than your own voice session after session helps break through the denial process. It's hard to keep up the pretense when four or five people within a circle are telling your own story in your own words with different names for the same characters; and when you join them in the chorus of "me, too," it strengthens your resolve when you go home to bank the fires burning out of control as the people who had it so good when you were acting addictively desperately attempt to undermine the good you're doing for yourself.

Because their lives are so dependent on the feelings and reactions of others, codependents have a strong need for control and a basic lack of trust. They are great at trying to figure out why things happen, and they believe once they understand why, they'll be fixed. Often they will present the results of their ruminations to their therapist and feel judged when the therapist looks confused.

The hardest thing codependents ever have to do is stop figuring out what everybody else wants and start figuring out what they want. You're the only one who knows what it's going to take to make you happy. If you want it, go for it. If's it's not right for you, God will stop you dead in your tracks—that's how you'll know what God's will is! But it will keep you in action instead of trying to make sense of everything *before* you take action.

Many new 12-step groups have formed around the

subject of codependence. You may want to find a group that meets regularly to discuss your problems of codependency.

ACTIVITIES FOR DAY NINETEEN

Assignment One: Serenity Prayer

"God grant me the serenity to accept the things I cannot change . . ."

List three situations in your life that you can't change and that you have difficulty accepting.

"The courage to change the things I can . . ."

List three situations in your life you are willing to change.

"And the wisdom to know the difference."

List three situations in your life that cause confusion because you are not sure whether you should accept them or try to change them.

Throughout the days to come, say the Serenity Prayer often and ask for help with the specific situations you have listed. God will hear you the first time. It's your own attention you need to get, and repeating the requests will eventually reach that part of you so resistant to change. In the process of writing these situations down, you will begin to clarify for yourself exactly what it is you need to do.

Assignment Two: Dysfunctional Family Systems

If you grew up in a dysfunctional family, you probably became codependent simply as a way to exist, and may find much in the following profile that you identify with. Put a check mark next to the things that apply to you. An adult child of a dysfunctional family often:

_____ 1. Has no concept of what "normal" is, and can be convinced that a dysfunctional situation is the norm, because there is no basis for comparison or healthy role models.

_____ 2. Has a difficult time following through. Projects get started but can't move from step to step to culmination. Having the right intention counts more than the ability to finish a task.

_____ 3. Devalues truth. Lies when there is no need to, and does so without guilt.

_____ 4. Is mercilessly judgmental of self and others.

_____ 5. Has a hard time having fun, never learned how to play, because life has always been so serious.

_____ 6. Is constantly seeking approval but cannot approve of self.

_____ 7. Overreacts to situations, particularly those over which there is no control, such as the weather or someone's lateness.

_____ 8. Has a twisted sense of loyalty. Will be excessively loyal to people who don't deserve it.

_____ 9. Acts on impulse, and once that impulse is triggered, must follow through in spite of fear of the consequences.

_____ 10. Is overly responsible. Often burns out, as the need for approval is so great that the ability to say no is diminished.

_____ 11. Has trouble delegating authority and working in cooperation with others. Learned to do it alone to avoid difficulties.

_____ 12. Seeks immediate gratification and has trouble delaying it, having grown up in an environment of emotional scarcity—"grab it now because if you wait it will be gone."

_____ 13. Becomes isolated and develops fear of authority figures.

_____ 14. Is frightened of criticism or the anger of others.

_____ 15. Sees self as a victim and is attracted to other victims.

_____ 16. Becomes addicted to a crisis atmosphere and will create chaos when things are going too smoothly.

_____ 17. Suppresses all feelings, good and bad, because it hurts too much to feel.

_____ 18. Reacts more than acts.

_____ 19. Doesn't know the difference between love and pity.

_____ 20. Develops compulsions, obsessions, addictions.

_____ 21. Is afraid of being alone, and willing to compromise too much to stay in a relationship.

If you checked off more than five of the above, you may have a problem with codependency. You may want to call the Codependency Helpline at 1-800-877-7675.

Assignment Three: Mixed Messages

Dysfunctional families are famous for sending out dual messages, especially when alcoholism is involved. The child is left to sort out the truth and invariably it comes out distorted. Here are some of those messages. See whether any of them apply to your situation:

1. "Everything is fine." Denial is strong in a dysfunctional family, but the tone of voice and general demeanor of the parent are in conflict with the words. The child recognizes this and can't account for the discrepancy. In the confusion it becomes difficult to sort out what is "fine" and what is not.

2. "Always tell me the truth." But the child soon learns that means the truth that the parent wants to hear. There is also the duality of the parent's lack of honesty. Eventually lying becomes the norm and truth unrecognizable.

3. "I promise you." The child of an alcoholic parent learns to live with broken promises, but is told that it is the intention, not the reality, that counts. To defend against disappointment, the child learns to have lowered or no expectations and to stop depending on others. The adult grows up isolating, overly self-sufficient, and unable to trust.

4. "I love you but . . ." It seems there's always a catch in a dysfunctional family, where love is conditional. Unconditional love is such a rarity that when the adult experiences it, that love doesn't feel real but is suspect.

If you identify with any of the above, you may have a problem with trust.

A DAY IN THE LIFE

Martha   *I'm supposed to write about what it means to me when someone breaks the rules. OK, my mother used to slap me across the face so hard I saw stars. I bet she gave me a concussion more than once, because sometimes my brain does funny things. I am thinking one thing, and then I'm thinking another, and there's a gap between where something went on but I don't know what. It just drives me crazy to think that part of my mind is not working. I'm afraid that I might say or do things I don't even know I'm saying or doing, and it's all because my mother used to hit me on the head with the back of her hand—WHAP—anywhere, any time, on the street, in the kitchen, and my dad did nothing to stop her. Nothing to stop her. No one did anything to stop her. She was that formidable. She was a tyrant. And she broke the rules! And no one did anything! My dad once promised me that he would make her stop. We were driving in his car, just the two of us, and he said he was going to take me and my brother away from her. Instead he left us behind and went away for good. And he PROMISED me that he would take me and my baby brother away—my mother hit him too, with that smack. She hit everybody. She even hit my dad, and none of us could ever hit back. It was the rule that no one could hit but her. So UNFAIR! She used to hurt my baby brother, and I just had to stand there and say nothing and do nothing, which is why now I have to. I have to I have to or I will go crazy and she will win my soul! I was always in a war to save my soul with her. She wanted that, too. She wanted to control everything. But I had my mind and she couldn't control that, and I told myself—I made a promise and I never break promises to myself—I told myself that when I grew up I would always fight for justice in these everyday things, like when a woman slaps a child on the street. You're damn right, I always speak up. And if that irritates people, well they can just go to hell! We're talking about my soul here.*

·

DAY TWENTY

Letting Go

As children, we wanted and deserved unconditional love and didn't get it. Consequently, we keep searching for it, and when it doesn't happen, we work harder at what doesn't work in the first place. As adults we have a choice. We can give and receive mature love. Here are four characteristics of that kind of healthy relationship.

One, it is open to being known to oneself and others. Both partners are willing to share their feelings and value honesty.

Two, it is accepting of oneself and the differences in others. Can someone take a different route home from the way you go without your getting anxious? Recognize your need for everyone to be the same as you and let it go. Acceptance includes past experiences. They happened. Now, how can they be used to make life better in the present?

Three, the healthy relationship is forgiving of the imperfections in oneself and others. It does not dwell on the guilt and shame of the past or on worry about the future.

Four, the healthy relationship allows for change, in perceptions, attitudes, and behavior. It encourages growth and is not afraid, even of the prospect of growing apart.

An addictive relationship makes a person feel consumed. A healthy relationship allows for individuality. In addictive love there is no definition of ego boundaries. Healthy belonging experiences both oneness with, and separateness from, a lover. Addictive love exhibits sadomasochism. Healthy loving brings out the best qualities in both partners. Addictive love fears letting go and does not allow for individual growth. Healthy love accepts endings and invites growth in the other partner. Psychological games, giving in order to get, and attempts to change the other are all part of addictive love. In a healthy relationship both giving and receiving are experienced in the same way, and there is no attempt to change or control the other partner.

Addictive lovers feel a need for each other to feel

complete. Healthy relationships encourage the self-sufficiency of both partners. The addictive lover demands and expects unconditional love and at the same time refuses commitment. Healthy love is grown-up and does not make infantile demands for unconditional love, and it welcomes commitment as a way of expressing love. Addictive love fears abandonment upon routine separation, looks to the other for affirmation and worth, and desires yet fears closeness. Healthy lovers have a high sense of self-worth, enjoy solitude, welcome closeness, and are able to risk vulnerability. The addictive lover attempts to take care of the other's feelings. Healthy love has boundaries that detach with love.

Mature lovers have conquered the question "Who am I?" They know what they want and need and what is important. In a healthy relationship the partners can appreciate their own individual talents, interests, creative potential, and pursuits. They know their closeness allows for individual difference. Commitment is characterized by desire, not only to give to the other, but to serve the other without expecting something in return. Mature lovers no longer need people in order to survive as they once did in childhood. They are aware that life is harsh at times, unfair at times, and yet continues to be good.

The healthy relationship is close but detached, which means not being distant or *un*involved but being truly grown-up and independent. It means being objective, but not indifferent; flexible, but not indecisive; firm, but not hard; wise, but not clever; patient, but not resigned; strong, but not overbearing; resolute, but not stubborn; compassionate, but not indulgent.

Detachment is profound love, wrapped in understanding and bound by courage. It helps you to live with serenity and fulfillment. It is a goal to strive for, because you deserve it!

ACTIVITIES FOR DAY TWENTY

Assignment One: Letting Go of a Destructive Relationship

If you are in an unhealthy relationship, or wonder if you are, draw a line down the center of a sheet of paper. At the top of the left-hand column write "What am I losing?" At the top of the right-hand column write "What am I gaining?" Under the left column write down all you are losing, including the qualities you admire in the person you love. Also write down all the qualities you don't admire. For example, maybe you are involved with someone who is a good listener, who is exciting, daring, intelligent, who stands up for what he believes in, but who is also jealous, blames others for his problems, complains a lot about things he can't change, and does not allow you enough privacy.

Imagine life without this person. What would you gain? Peace of mind? The chance to find a more compatible mate? More personal freedom? Take the time to fully explore your future potential. You might find you *don't* have much to gain from losing this person. If that is so, then maybe you had better reconsider whether this relationship is truly destructive, or whether it can be improved with some help. On the other hand, you might find there is much to gain from letting go of this person, and that may provide you with the resolve you need.

If you have decided you must let go of this relationship, take a look at your list again. The positive aspects you wrote down are the qualities you want to look for in someone else. The negatives are what you want to avoid in someone else. There is never one person on earth for anyone. The world is full of millions of people, many of them engaged in the same search you are. If you seek out the qualities you value, you are likely to find them.

Assignment Two: Face It; Trace It; Erase It

Write in your diary the ways in which you have been spiritually, emotionally, and sexually violated. Describe how the violation made you feel and how it affects your behavior today. Discuss the subtle ways in which a person can be violated, such as being held in a sexual way when you were expecting a friendly hug (physical), or being told that enjoying your body will result in Hell and damnation (spiritual), or having your accomplishments ignored or devalued (emotional).

Read what you have written aloud, as if the person or persons who violated you were in the room.

Assignment Three: Forgiveness

Forgiveness does not require that you tell the people who did you harm that you are forgiving them. It is a selfish act done only for yourself so you can feel better. In no way does it condone what they did. Rather, it is a conscious decision to surrender your feelings. Anger, resentment, and hate are luxuries we food addicts can't afford, for they will cause us to relapse back into our addiction.

Forgiveness is a release of feelings: you must feel them, deal with them, and give them up, so the space they took up can be filled with love. You don't have to forgive everyone at once, only as you can. When you want hate less than love, you will be willing to make the exchange.

Forgiveness is the key to loving yourself. If you can choose not to forgive and hold on to your pain, you can also choose to let go, for there are two sides to everything. Mary A. Dombroski, Ph.D., has developed a helpful acronym for the forgiveness process called ADDS:

> *Awareness* means crossing the threshold of denial and acknowledging that the wrongs inflicted happened and that they hurt.

> *Discovering* means sharing those feelings with others, for communicating them makes them real. You have been carrying the burden of your secret, and sharing that secret does away with it just as a sunrise does away with night. Once a secret is shared, it loses its power and becomes real.

> *Decision* means a willingness to let go. Holding on to the discovery will give it power again. Detaching from it is a choice to make for health.

> *Serenity* is the healing gift of forgiveness.

When people don't forgive, it's about false pride and being judgmental. Humility is about forgiving. It's learning to come to everyone with love, even people who have wronged you. It doesn't matter what people do. It's more important what you do. I know it hurts and I'm not negating the emotional or physical pain if you've been injured by someone, but I think to have dignity we have to come to everyone out of love. That's why forgiveness is so important. Without it you can't come from love.

Draw up a list of three people who have hurt you. Write each one a letter, describing in detail the harm they did to you and how it has affected your life. Describe the feelings you still carry about their deeds. Take each letter, crumble it in a ball, put it in a sink, and set fire to it. As it burns, say, "I forgive you." When the letters are nothing but ashes, dispose of them, clean the sink, and get on with the business of living.

Assignment Four: Visualization for Forgiveness

Sit comfortably and quiet your mind as you have been practicing. One by one, visualize the people who harmed you as a child as little children themselves. Focus on their faces and note whether they are sad. If they are, ask them what they need. Then reach in and embrace those little children. Tell them that you love them and are setting them free.

A DAY IN THE LIFE

Chuck *I forgive you, Mom. You did the best you could. You were in the thrall of your addiction, and I know what a powerful grip that is now. You did what you could to give us what we needed. You loved to buy food for us even though we never all sat down to the table at the same time, our life was so chaotic. But you wanted to care for me. I remember when you would sneak into my room after Dad beat me, and you would read me a bedtime story as if nothing had happened. And then you'd tell me how I was going to go to college. And I went to college. You tried as hard as you could, and no one was there to help you like there is here. No one ever said to you, "Do you have a problem? Is something troubling you?" No one said, "Can I help you?" You were caught in a prison, and you stayed there until you died. Poor, beloved mom who brought me into the world. I miss you, I forgive you, and I am a good father in your name. It is my way of forgiving you, to be a good parent. It proves to me that there is good and bad in everyone, and if I'm partly good it's because you and Dad were, too. Nothing is all black and white. People are good, bad, but mostly in between. I just am, me, Chuck, an average guy who gets a big kick out of life. Tomorrow my wife comes. I'm as nervous as a teenager on a first date.*

•

DAY TWENTY-ONE

Protecting the Spirit

When we were children we were playful and spontaneous. What happened? Some of us have forgotten how to play because of messages we learned about how we "should" or "ought" to be. But the child we were is still alive within us, and we can teach it new messages. In gratitude, that child will come out and teach the adult in us how to be playful, creative, and spontaneous. But first that child of yours has to learn to trust you. He has been abused or neglected by you. How many times have you scolded yourself out loud? Your inner child takes that to heart and feels wounded. She may be wondering if anyone will ever come and rescue her. If you want to rescue your inner child, you need to remember that you have not done much over the years to inspire trust.

We speak to that inner child through visualization, as children respond more readily to pictures than words. For that reason, this explanation is short today, like a child's attention span, so you can go right to work on communicating with your child in pictures.

ACTIVITIES FOR DAY TWENTY-ONE

Assignment One: Visualization

Choose a time when you can be alone and uninterrupted. Find a photograph of yourself as a child, preferably one that is full face, in which you can see your eyes. If you have a record or tape of environmental music of ocean sounds, play it softly in the background, or play some beautiful and soothing music of your choice.

Sit comfortably with the photograph on your lap and begin meditating the way you have been practicing. When your mind is quieted, pick up the photograph of yourself and focus on that small face. Look directly into the eyes of that little child. Then close your eyes and see the face in your mind. See what your inner child is wearing. Notice the setting: Is your child hiding? You may have to coax it to come forward. Is it sitting or standing? What kind of expression is on its face? As you see that child, allow yourself to have compassion in your mind's eye, and then step into the scene and put your arms around your child. Let it know you're there and that it's important to you. Now pick up your child and speak soothingly. Ask your child, "What did you need to hear but never did?" When you hear the answer, tell your child that now. Let your child talk to you freely about its pain, and when it has told you everything it needs to tell you, ask what it needs.

When you hear the answer, give your child what it needs at once, either emotionally or symbolically. Then take your child's hand and go for a walk by the ocean. Enjoy the feel of the sand beneath your feet and the breeze on your cheeks. Listen to your child the way you wanted to be listened to when you were little. Let your child know how much you love it and that you will always be there.

Assignment Two: A Letter from Your Spirit

Using your nondominant hand, write a letter from your spirit to your adult self, expressing whatever feelings come to mind. With the dominant hand, write as an adult to your inner child, acknowledging the child's pain. Begin to nurture and comfort it. You and your child may begin a dialogue, or you may be more comfortable with letters.

The nondominant hand creates a pipeline to the inner child, circumventing the mind-set of the adult. You may want to use it whenever you feel out of touch with your child, or when you are feeling good about yourself and want to send it an extra dose of comfort and love.

Assignment Three: The Nurturing Parent

Your spirit needs plenty of nurturing, to make up for what you needed long ago and never got. Take a big sheet of paper and with crayons or colored felt-tipped pens, draw a big picture of your nurturing parent—holding a balloon, smiling and loving and warm and constant. Now write inside the balloon, comic strip style, the messages you longed to hear when you were growing up. Examples: "How proud I am of you." "I love you just the way you are." "You are so beautiful." Attach the drawing to a wall, the back of a door, or another place where you can see it frequently.

A DAY IN THE LIFE

Jenny   I'm still weak from all the crying my mom and I did. The session just opened the floodgates. It was so good for her—I know. Stop right there. I was so good for me to see and hear her cry and rage and sob and have strong emotions! I have never in all my life, up until today, seen my mother do more than dab her eyes at funerals and sad movies. She is one angry woman. I couldn't get angry back at her though, in spite of how much I needed to do it—still need to do it. How could she have been so unconscious of the fact that I had feelings? I couldn't do it because I now see that my mom has always been unconscious that she has feelings. It just felt so good when we cried and sobbed in each others' arms over how we felt about the breakup of the family, and how jealous we were of "the replacement," as mom called her (I was shocked!), and how hard it was for us to move clear across the country to get away *from the pain of being near him and our old apartment and neighborhood and all, and then start a new life. We were so totally unprepared for what faced us!*

I feel so light now. I feel as if I could float right out of here and scan the globe and float back in again if I wanted to. Or I could sing like an opera singer or do a cartwheel, all if I wanted to. I am just not quite sure I am ready to do all those things yet. I just want to sit here and feel the relief. Oh, Mama, why can't you go out and get yourself a life? What are you afraid of???

•

7

Week Four: In Recovery

The changes in Chuck, Martha, and Jenny are now markedly observable. Martha has been the most deeply moved spiritually. She confided to Bob, her primary therapist, that there had been an angel in her room. Her deeply buried spirit has received a message that it can break free of her bonds, and that knowledge has caused a volcanic disruption of her surface behavior, increasing her need to control to the maximum. The patients protested her tyrannizing at the community meeting, and Martha fled from the room. Her wails penetrated the floor as she banished herself like a vanquished Napoleon. Martha is in a struggle for her life, and everyone knows it. That acknowledgment makes it safe for her to keep going, not in a struggle, but in the decision to stop struggling.

Chuck has also made deep changes. He is looking at his need to be a good person as a twisted revenge against his parents, and now that the forgiveness process has begun, he realizes he is a good person already and doesn't "have" to be anything more than he is for other people. What he has to focus on is being good to himself. Chuck is also excited over the impending visit of his wife. He says, "It will be a kind of second honeymoon after this is all over."

When Jenny's pretty, youthful mother came in for family group, it was obvious that the mother and daughter loved each other very much and yet could not find a way to express their true emotions. Having feelings was simply a foreign idea to them. Their genteel upbringing did not allow for that kind of expression. They both had much difficulty finding words for how they felt, as if they had just learned the basics of a foreign language. But when Jenny began to cry with deep, wrenching sobs while telling her mother how she felt when told of her parents' separation, her mother took her in her arms and held her daughter for a long time and they cried together. It was not necessary for them to express their deep feelings in words at that moment. The experience was particularly healing for Jenny, who had wanted her mother's comfort and acknowledgment in just such a way all these years. Jenny's mother left determined to seek help for the depression she has suffered for twenty years since the breakup of her marriage to a man she said she still deeply loves.

The goal of the last week of treatment is to lay down the behavior changes that have been made, to fortify them by repetition, to make way for more breakthroughs, and to prepare for bringing this new way of living home.

After twenty-one days of nourishing the body with fresh whole foods and cleansing it of all harmful and addictive substances, you too will be quite literally a different person. We coexist with our addictions so long that they feel like the norm. But the absence of high-fat foods and refined sugar has quieted the craving to feed your emotions, and in that silence you can think, feel, or just be. You also have a new concept of energy—not the cycle of rushes and exhaustion that caffeine causes. One person had beaten rhythms with her fingers and toes for years, unable to will herself to stop. Once her body was free from caffeine, the "involuntary" movements stopped of their own accord.

As beneficial as the effect of the *absence* of harmful substances, is the nourishment of the food you are providing, which has now reached the cellular level. You hum like an expensive car. When the only thing that goes into your mouth is fresh, pure, and whole, you are giving yourself nutrients that may not even have been discovered yet! You are eating like a hunter—gatherer in the time before food preservation and all the other changes of modern society. Eating like our ancestors gives us the nourishment we need without having to give much thought to exactly what we eat, and in time, how much we eat, because the body will once again have become a smoothly running organism telling what it needs when it needs it. You can't get enough of what you don't need, goes the axiom. But you *can* get enough of what your body needs and it will return the favor by determining how *much* it needs by itself, without your conscious participation. Imagine the peace of that.

I am sure that if you have adopted the food preparation tips I provided early in the book and are using fresh, whole food, you are now enjoying eating sensations you forgot existed. You will have rediscovered the sweetness of fresh fruit and the superior flavor of virgin olive oil over the corn or soy oils used in prepared salad dressings. You will have discovered how wonderful a puree-thickened meal can be. Because all these new sensations are good tasting and good for the body, they are truly satisfying.

Another dramatic difference by the twenty-second day of recovery is what exercise brings. Suddenly you slip your pants on without tugging. Your legs and arms are more shapely. If you have been exercising for half an hour each day, breaking into a sweat for at least fifteen minutes, your body will have taken over by now in the motivation department. It is a much studied phenomenon that a new habit can be laid down in twenty-one days of repetition. While your mind hems and haws, your body just moves its legs and does it. You are now in a place where you don't have to struggle to exercise anymore. It is another source of peace that lies deep. We *want* to move our bodies. It is the natural way. And our bodies love to do what they were so wondrously well designed to do. Exercise's benefits to the body are like those of eating fresh food: a slow and steady and increasing sense of well-being. It is the nature of things to grow toward the light. You are now in the fullness of that light.

DAY TWENTY-TWO

The "Real You" Emerges

You are what you are what you are, if you can just step out of your way. With enough letting go, that positive and creative human being will be set free. In the course of recovery, you have let go of the defense mechanisms you have been using to protect your real self, letting go on faith that you were doing the right thing. You have let go of your past and reframed your early childhood messages, acting to change them instead of struggling with them. You have let go of the roles you play in lieu of who you really are. You have let go of grief and loss of love from the past, allowing negative emotions to surface, and you have accepted your limitations, letting go of the need for perfection and your magical thinking. You have let go of your family and personal secrets and practiced forgiveness. You have identified painful underlying issues, taken care of unfinished business, and allowed yourself to be helpless and powerless, vulnerable and without defenses.

You have let go of your isolation and begun to bond with others, and you have practiced relaxation techniques to reduce stress and fear. You have taken risks by acting assertively and expressed feelings in effective and appropriate ways. You have made choices in spite of your fears and built trust in yourself and others. You have established boundaries and defended them, learning communications skills that allow you to say what you mean and mean what you say, to respond instead of react, and to share instead of tell. You have developed healthy eating patterns and rituals to change your negative thought patterns to positive ones. You have learned to hug, laugh, and feel. You have become real, and in the end, that is all that matters.

You have become a spiritual being, translucent, open, someone who lives in the here and now, who dares to be spontaneous, who is glad to help others. You know you are not your body but God's child, and you love who that is. You love who you are and want to claim your power. You're confident. You respond, not react, and that empowers the Real Me.

Love does not fail you when you don't get it. It fails you when you don't give it. Love does not guarantee popularity. Love requires that I say what I believe and do what I consider right. As addicts, we demand love and treat people or allow others to treat us as things—objects for love. But real love allows people room to breathe, to have their own identity, to be responsible for themselves, sometimes loving the person enough to let go.

Real love is passion, commitment, and intimacy. Passion is the powerful force in nature that draws two people together for procreation, but it will not last beyond a few days or weeks if that is all there is to the connection. Commitment is also necessary, the glue that keeps a relationship going after the initial excitement is over. But people sometimes stay together out of commitment alone, without experiencing real love. That needs a third element, intimacy. As you have learned, you can't be intimate with another until you know and love yourself. You are now ready for real love. You can choose whom you will become intimate with rather than settle for anyone out of fear and desperation. Your repressed sexuality, sensuality, and creativity will start to flow, and you will become exciting to others.

Father Booth likes to draw a triangle to show what true spirituality is. One side is emotions, the second body, the third mind, all encompassed in Spirit. He disagrees with the concept that the human being is mind, body, and spirit, and so do I, for it isolates spirituality from body and mind. Especially in dealing with eating disorders and their abuse of the body, it's important that people start to love and take care of their bodies as a spiritual entity. The sum of all our parts is our spirituality. God lives in us and other people in a state of tangibility. This kind of spirituality couldn't be further from the kind of religion that imprisons the spirit, that molests people's minds with ideas that sex is dirty, that menstruation is "the curse," that you can't go to God without a priest, that everything we enjoy, God is against. It's staggering how many obese people attend religious centers where spirituality is abused.

I believe you become like the God you believe in, so if you believe in a God of anger, you'll be angry; in a God who judges, you'll judge. But if your God is loving, accepting, and caring, you will become those things, too.

ACTIVITIES FOR DAY TWENTY-TWO

Assignment One: Body Image

Ask yourself:

1. Whose body would you most want yours to look like? Why?

2. How do you feel about your body? What features do you like best about yourself? What features do you like least?

3. Close your eyes and take time to create scenes of yourself in the body you would like to have in the following situations—an office party, playing volleyball at a picnic, having sex. How would you move, talk, and envision others seeing you? See how you interact with the opposite sex.

Assignment Two: Re-create: A Meditation

The Real You does not have to be created from scratch—it has been there all along, in a disconnected state. The Real You was disconnected, not so much by the trauma itself, but by the defensive patterns developed as a result of that trauma. The Real You had detached itself in order to survive the pain: by disconnecting, the Real You buried itself and no longer felt anything at all. The negativity of addiction further blocks connection with the Real You, but believe me, IF YOU CAN MAKE A CONNECTION, NOTHING WILL STOP YOU FROM FULFILLING YOUR SELF-DETERMINED DESTINY.

This meditation is on making that connection. Reflect, in a state of quietude, on what it would mean to base your relationships on values, beliefs, and integrity instead of your old needs to control, please, or isolate. Reflect on how the re-creation that takes place once you are connected to your spirit will bring a new energy to everything in your life. You have a right to that re-creation and to the "feel good" endorphins it will bring.

Assignment Three: Where Your Spirit Can Take You: A Visualization

A wise philosopher once said, "First you dream it." If there is something you desire, a goal you have wanted to reach for some time, a change you want to make in your environment or circumstances, be grateful that you have a burning desire. Sometimes I think the hardest part of recovery is getting people to pay attention to their desires—what they really want to do with their life.

Imagine that desire is a map. You find it unexpectedly one day while looking for something else. WITHOUT DELAY you prepare for your departure, taking along only what you need. You take your car in for a major tune-up. You take care of all the necessary details, and then you get in the car and pull out of town. Your heart is racing—at last! We're on the road!

Your map is at your side, on the seat of the car. You come to a crossroads and pull over in a shady rest stop and spread the map on the hood of the car. Oh yes, that's how to get there. No hurry though. Enjoy the ride. Take the scenic route. Maybe it will take you a little longer to get there, but it will be well worth the experience.

And so there you are. You open your eyes. Now what?

A DAY IN THE LIFE

Martha   They asked me to describe the angel in my room. I am a cynical woman. I become angry, angry, angry, all the time angry. My mother was angry and so she hit me. She believed she had the right, and her belief couldn't be shaken. She thought she was like God—she made me so she could do what she wanted to with me. And in my mind today I am still hitting myself. I can't shake my mother's belief either, and that's what's keeping me stuck. Should this beating be going on or shouldn't it? Do I deserve to be beaten or don't I? For years I have been driving myself nuts with this question, but I couldn't even put it into words until the angel came into my room. I was really giving it to myself good after the community meeting when I was humiliated and criticized. I was reading one of the books here that we're supposed to read, but I kept beating myself *up in my mind. I can see the stick now and a shadowy creature above me hitting and hitting, again and again. I felt the blows on my head and shoulders, and I couldn't crouch enough. And then the angel was there. I could sense its wings hovering around my cowering shoulders, and I didn't see but somehow felt this beautiful being with wings, and it was standing above the creature with the stick who kept beating me. And in that moment, I realized the angel had stopped the beating. It didn't call out; it just kept hovering above the creature with the stick until there was no more creature. It dissolved. All that was left was a feeling of being safe and a warm sensation inside me. Somehow I feel that angel has been hovering nearby all along; I just never paid attention to it. I don't know why. I think it has something to do with having to control everything. I knew there was help, but I was not willing to let go of the control. I can let go now. I could never stop the beating, but the angel could.*

If anyone reads this they will think I am nuts. But then who cares what they think? You know what? I don't care what they think! I don't care what any of you think. And that makes me glad.

•

DAY TWENTY-THREE

Protecting the Spirit: Establishing Boundaries

Boundaries are like a kaleidoscope. They refract the world so you can observe patterns instead of being a victim. I once had a patient who said she couldn't say no to a man under any circumstances. Lacking boundaries to that extent is a form of paralysis. Food, alcohol, and other mood-altering substances create artificial boundaries. Once you abstain from them, you have to learn to create real boundaries in order to feel comfortable in the world.

Boundaries are essential to successful relationships. You can't connect with another unless you are a separate person. Many food addicts come from enmeshed families where members are extensions of each other. If you had thoughts and ideas that were different from those of your relatives, did they feel slighted and offended? If they did, you were not allowed to be separate from them. In such a system, intimacy feels like drowning because your individualism goes down the drain.

People who were not allowed to make boundaries when they were children have a hard time creating them as adults. They guess what others feel, or make people guess what they're feeling. They indulge in magical thinking and endure negative relationships by keeping a fantasy alive that everything is fine.

Creating a boundary means paying attention to your level of discomfort. Addicts are accustomed to all-or-nothing thinking and are not aware of graduals. How close is too close? How much is too much? The only way to determine where those boundaries are is to pay attention to your discomfort level. For instance, if someone is standing too close to you, do you step back? What if that person approaches you again? Will you end up being backed into a corner, or can you say, "When you stand this close to me, I feel uncomfortable"? If you can't make that statement because you don't want the other person to be uncomfortable (although it's all right for you to be!), then you have trouble establishing boundaries.

When people who have difficulty with boundaries do finally manage to establish one and it's crossed, they are really vulnerable. Yet, it's the rare perpetual trespasser who doesn't try, almost as if a boundary line were a challenge. Try not to take it personally. Think of it as a test, and pay attention to how you feel. Your discomfort will only increase unless you reestablish your limits.

If the only way you can have a relationship with someone is by tolerating his or her crossing your line, you're not being valued as a person. If you're told "I think you're too sensitive" when you define a boundary, your answer is a resolute "My problem is I haven't been sensitive enough."

You may be surprised at the resistance you will meet when you begin establishing boundaries, especially with those who previously felt free to roam wherever they pleased. For instance, if you tell someone what's important to you and he or she brushes you aside, as if what you said was of no consequence, take note and make a quick exit. This person is not someone to get close to. Or if a person tries to alter what's true for you by saying, "It's really not so bad" or "It's nothing compared to my situation" or "Don't worry about it. Trust me," it's boundary city. My criterion for trust is simply, someone hears what I say and honors it. If I make a statement about myself and someone replies with a statement that begins with "You should" or "You're too," he or she has violated my barrier. People can make statements about themselves all they like, but when they make a statement about me, my best interest is in jeopardy.

Assertiveness doesn't guarantee you are correct, or that you will get respect or what you want, but it establishes you as assertive. It sends out the message "Don't tread on me" to those who make a habit of treading on others, deliberately or otherwise. You will recognize who they are when you start paying attention to your body. You will feel discomfort and make a deft getaway.

You are also giving an important message to that little kid you carry around inside—that you are taking care of business, that you matter, that you aren't afraid of a little discomfort to define who you are, and that you don't need the approval of others because you have your own.

People without boundaries are afraid of intimacy because they fear engulfment, for good reason. People keep getting too close, make too many demands. But once you feel safe behind the boundaries you have drawn for yourself, you can establish true intimacy with others.

ACTIVITIES FOR DAY TWENTY-THREE

Assignment One: Boundary Alert

In the course of the next three days, pay extra attention to the clues your body gives that a boundary is being crossed. If you respond by feeling anxious, fearful, angry, or trapped, write a memo to yourself, literally or mentally, depending on the situation. At the first opportunity, explore why your body sounded the alarm. What did the other person do or say that triggered your response? Script a "when you . . . I feel . . ." response. Say it aloud, looking in a mirror. Your spirit will get the message that you are working on protecting it. Pay attention to what you see as you talk into the mirror.

Assignment Two: Boundary Changes

When you set new boundaries, you are bound to get a reaction. That is why they need to be clearly defined. Remember, without the artificial boundary of your mood-altering substances, you are going to feel incredibly vulnerable unless the new ones are firmly in place.

Select three people in your life with whom you are setting new boundaries. Describe how the old boundary has been—unpredictable, enmeshed, chaotic, etc. Describe how the new boundary is defined. Be precise. Pay particular attention to what is now off limits: At what point is this person now trespassing where before he or she was free to go? This is the point of conflict: denying someone access where they were previously free to roam. This is where the difficulty will come. Prepare yourself: Script your answers. Write down three responses to an insistence that your boundary be crossed. Say them to yourself frequently. Soon you will come to believe that you have the right to this new boundary, and then you will defend it without the slightest difficulty! Entitlement will show you exactly why and how, without that old awful feeling.

A DAY IN THE LIFE

Chuck   *What a surprise my wife was today in the group session. She was so angry! I had no idea she had such strong feelings in her. When she yelled it was like she had laryngitis—couldn't quite make the sounds. But the tears were real. In our private session Jean told me things that knocked my socks off, like being sexually abused by her brothers, and because of the abuse never really enjoying sex with me. That blows me away. All these years I thought we had had this great sex life, and here it was all this time just her trying to please me! She needs to come here. She's got a whole life's load of anger to discharge—anger at the kids for taking advantage of her, anger at me for not being able to guess how she really feels, anger at her father and mother for not protecting her, anger at her brothers. She has been eating her anger—literally—all those crunchy potato chips and hard candies and giant pretzels she loves. By the time the session was through, I was speechless. But I've got a lot to say to her, and a lot to convey to her that doesn't require words. I think now that she has finally talked about the sexual abuse, we can get closer in bed. Before it was always the two of us and her secret.*

This whole revelation has had a great, but strange impact on me, I guess because it's new for me to be there for a person but not to feel required to jump in and solve all her problems. From observing the people here who have been sexually abused, especially the ones who were abused by a family member, I know that the damage is profound in terms of the course their life takes, and that the healing is a long process. Trust has been violated, and when it comes down to it, what is more valuable in a relationship than trust? I feel my trust in my wife has been shaken because of her deception. I mean, what a good liar she is! I want to make some inquiries so we can get help together or separately, whatever we need. We need to heal and work our problems out together. I have so much hope.

·

DAY TWENTY-FOUR

Relationships

The quality of our relationships reveals whether we have resolved our unfinished business or are still struggling. If we can't have healthy, satisfying relationships, it's a clue that we still are disconnected. Our disconnected selves engage in relationships as if they were in a field of battle—protecting and defending—only now and then letting down our guard. Being wounded in an intimate relationship is the deepest wound of all, because we thought we were safe and let our defenses down only to be hurt. It's why some people give up on intimacy altogether.

But our relationships cannot be otherwise when we are disconnected from our spirits. In the disconnected state, we numb ourselves to the present and remain frozen in the past. If we do allow ourselves to become involved with anybody, we use the relationship to act out unresolved conflicts of the past. We don't see our relationships for what they are or could be; instead, they are reenactments or desperate attempts to resolve our unfinished business.

If you are not currently in a relationship, it may be a good idea to spend a year without getting emotionally entangled with anyone. That gives you time to sort out the past and the present, and "work through" what you have been discovering about yourself. You will be able to develop new patterns and new attitudes about people; you'll have time to focus on nourishing your spirit.

Like recovery from major surgery, early spiritual recovery is a time to take care and to heal slowly. Emerging from that time of healing, you will be able to have relationships by connecting with other loving spirits. Because you are all reconnected and can allow the Real You to emerge, your relationships will be enhanced and you'll experience what real intimacy is all about.

ACTIVITIES FOR DAY TWENTY-FOUR

Assignment One: Letting in: A Meditation

The idea that physical intimacy is a surrendering scares some people. They don't like not being in control. Instead, reflect on the image of letting in. Reflect on the trust that gesture requires. Trust is really what love is all about. It's not about fear of rejection; it's not about excitement and danger. Love is the anticipation and acceptance of another person. Love is opening your heart, your soul, and letting another touch your spirit.

Imagine yourself experiencing that trust. Imagine how your body would dissolve into that trust, to merge with another, to experience love, caring, and intimacy.

Assignment Two: Eight Reasons Not to Have Sex

1. To settle arguments
2. For companionship
3. To relieve guilt
4. To express anger
5. To humiliate your partner
6. To deal with jealousy
7. To confirm sexual identity
8. To relieve loneliness

For each of these eight reasons, describe a setting outside of sex where the issues could be appropriately expressed. Which of the reasons do you identify with the most?

A DAY IN THE LIFE

Jenny   I want to write about this little girl who believed in fairy tales, who would wait by the window for her daddy to come home. Father and daughter were so close, I bet that little kid knew in her bones long before the big announcement came that he was leaving. And she's still inside of me today, still waiting by the window in the living room with the poster of Jimi Hendrix on the wall in that wonderful old apartment in Fort Greene, Brooklyn. She's still back in those "fairy-tale" days of my childhood when my parents took me to demonstrations and neighborhood meetings, food cooperatives, and to my grandparents' farm down south every summer. It wasn't that my childhood was ideal. Bad things were going on, my parents told me so. That was why we were in the demonstrations—to stop the bad things going on in the neighborhood. But the fairy-tale part is believing that world would go on forever, that we would always sit down to the table together, or sit on the couch and watch TV for a while just before bed-

time. I had so many connections then and they have all been broken, connections to my neighborhood as well as my parents. Everyone on the block knew who I was, and all the mothers kept one eye out for me, just as my mom did for the other kids. I also had my relatives—a huge bunch of people who made holidays such a hectic but joyous time. I was an only child, but believe me, I was never lonely. No wonder I never wanted to leave that childhood world. It was pretty idyllic, given the circumstances.

The number one valuable thing I've learned here is that I'm not that ten-year-old today, although I carry her spirit inside me as delicately as I would a rare and beautiful butterfly. I have discovered the Real Me here, Jennifer Louise, and I am astonished to discover other people really want to get to know that person. Not just the married men looking for an affair, but real people wanting to make real connections.

I don't ever want to go back to being that sad, lonely little girl sitting on the window seat with her dolls and her books, waiting. There is a place for me, but it is not back there, frozen in time and space. It is here. Wherever I am is my place, and the real me is in it, solid. And this me is not alone anymore. The people I have come to know in the rooms up and down the hall are just plain people. We all bleed. We all came in here desperate and suffering. We have learned the joy and relief of being real. I discovered my mother in this place, and she discovered me. We hugged each other, and we were flesh and blood. I will always remember that warm feeling, that comfort, and how I had always yearned for her closeness even more than I had yearned for my daddy to come home.

The second most valuable thing I have learned here: my real motivations. I went into engineering because I wanted to be in a man's world, I wanted to be surrounded by them and that's a fact. I figured that out my freshman year. But I also worshipped the certitude of math. There was no magic in it, for I had learned the lesson of believing in magic when as a child, I made all those wishes and magic spells trying to get my parents back together, and they didn't work. Math was all fact. With it, there were no surprises once you understood the equation. It never betrayed my trust like people did. I was lucky. It turned out I loved my choice of profession, but I am glad to admit to my other motivations because it feels good. I'm translucent, and I have nothing to hide—even the weak parts of me—because I understand the weaknesses and where they come from. I know they don't make up who I am.

The third gift of treatment: my roommate Peggy. She came in here fighting for her life. I could feel her spirit leave her and come floating above the curtains around her bed. I prayed for her those first few days. She said she heard me, although I didn't say my prayers out loud. I could feel when Peggy decided to live. I was there when Peggy began to grieve for her mother, who was killed in a car crash when she was six years old, and for her husband, who was killed in the same way two years ago. That was when Peggy slid into chronic depression.

My ability to be there for Peggy is like a gift. Recovery is give and take. The thing about Peggy is she gives back. Martha just takes. Peggy gives back in so many little ways all the time, like with her attitude. She can make a funny joke on the spot about a toothbrush. She just sees the humorous side of everything. She says to Martha, "Martha darlin', you do it your way, I'll do it mine," and defuses her on the spot. In fact, she laughs! We both humor Martha when she gets fixated on trifles. We call her on her need to control and respond with love and ask her what she really needs. We are respectful of her. We believe her about the angel because ever since then, she's been a different woman. Now when she goes into her old Martha act, it's like it's involuntary. But she's shedding it little by little like an old worn coat you don't want to wear anymore.

•

DAY TWENTY-FIVE

Step Study: Steps Four Through Twelve

The Twelve Steps are a way of life and require action. They are not read so much as worked. The Step Study in this book is only a basic introduction to them, for they become more meaningful as you progress in recovery. Some people spend years working on Step One. Others come into the program ready to work on Step Twelve! There are no deadlines to meet. People proceed at the pace they feel they are ready for, although many in the program use one step a year as a guideline.

In Steps One through Three, we admitted our powerlessness, came to believe in a power greater than ourselves, and turned over our will to this higher power.

The following is a synopsis of Steps Four to Twelve, as an introduction, and to prepare you for what lies ahead. The beauty of the Twelve Steps is that they focus on you. They are concerned only with your own growth, for the sole purpose of making you "happy, joyous, and free." They are not dogma, only the most practical of applications of basic human principles to one's daily life.

By the time people have worked through Step Three, they have made a commitment to the program. They have acknowledged their powerlessness, that their lives have become unmanageable, that there is a power greater than themselves that they have tapped into, and a need to relinquish their wills to this higher power.

Until the results of surrender are experienced—when help does arrive as promised, through other people, and begins to work, restoring sanity to your life—the steps beyond the third will seem insurmountable. But power comes from tapping into this great resource that is available to all of us willing to surrender our wills, and it gives us an entirely new outlook on life. Suddenly, it *is* possible to change, and the energy required for change is there, in abundance. So read these steps with the realization that there is outside help in doing them. Otherwise you will feel too much is required. And don't *think* too much about them. Action is the key to this program, one day at a time. Miracles are common, but they do not just happen.

Step Four

"Made a searching and fearless moral inventory of ourselves."

People recoil from this step. Suddenly they are hit with the realization that this program is going to require them to change, and they don't think they're ready. But without change, there is nothing. Pain isn't about change, it's about resisting change. The catharsis of the first three steps—when one experiences the great relief and joy of discovering there is help in the universe and that life's problems need not be dealt with in isolation—is not enough for recovery. Change begins within, with a strong searchlight beamed inward.

Inventory is not a critical evaluation. It is an assessment. It examines assets, finds out what there is enough of, too much of, and what is lacking in order to conduct business. A moral inventory is an examination of needs. When you are ready to take the Fourth Step, you will list your assets first and then take a look at your character defects, the things about you that cause negative consequences, and be ready to acknowledge them fully.

Step Five

"Admitted to God, to ourselves, and to another human being the exact nature of our wrongs."

Step Five is a catharsis. It does not result in an overnight change, but it does bring the relief of having no more secrets to bear alone. In the process of accepting ourselves, with all our defects, our acceptance of others grows. We no longer expect perfection of anyone, especially ourselves.

Step Six

"Were entirely ready to have God remove all these defects of character."

This step is not as simple as it seems. We are secretly fond of many of our character defects and don't really want to give them up. The power God has to remove these defects is experienced at the point of surrender, when the insane craving for a mood-altering substance is lifted out. The miracle of that prepares us, although the removal of our character defects is more gradual and ongoing than the lifting of our craving for food.

Step Seven

"Humbly asked Him to remove our shortcomings."

Humility is always difficult. To most people it equates with weakness, but it is nothing more than a desire to seek and do God's will. If we became humble, our behavior will gradually and remarkably change.

Step Eight

"Made a list of all persons we had harmed, and became willing to make amends to them all."

The person at the top of our lists should be ourselves, and learning to make amends to ourselves first will help us make amends to the others we have harmed, out of fear, resentment, sex, and pride. The inventory of Step Eight is even more difficult than that of Step Four, because it forces us to confront our deeds, and the pain we have caused, something we have probably worked hard to deny. The humility required of us in the previous step prepares us.

Step Nine

"Made direct amends to such people wherever possible, except when to do so would injure them and others."

Sometimes making amends is easy. A child is listened to, a spouse is treated with respect, a debt is paid. Apologies are often in order, but amends are about action more than words. Behavior change means more than the most eloquent plea for forgiveness. In certain situations direct amends are not possible. The person harmed may have died. Someone who loved you may be in a new relationship, and hearing from you would reopen rather than heal a wound. Or a spouse might be greatly harmed to hear about your extramarital adventures. Each compensation must be carefully evaluated, but when it is appropriate, screwing up one's courage and being forthright without getting excessively remorseful is the way to do it.

Step Ten

"Continued to take personal inventory and when we were wrong promptly admitted it."

One of the characteristics of people who have been in a 12-step program for a long time is their willingness to admit they are wrong. It is such a rare thing in this world that they stand out as special. Admitting it promptly is possible if a daily inventory is taken, for carrying around the knowledge of a wrong committed against someone is poisonous, and it must be discharged. It's a lot easier to be ignorant of the wrongs we do, for awareness of them carries the responsibility of action. The benefit of acting in an esteemable way is worth the humility required by this step. We can be glad we are who we are, because we live honestly. We have nothing to hide, and nothing to be ashamed of, even our imperfections, for we readily admit them.

Step Eleven

"Sought through prayer and meditation to improve our conscious contact with God as we understood Him, praying only for knowledge of His will for us and the power to carry that out."

Life becomes remarkably simple by the Eleventh Step. We don't need to make agonizing decisions about what we should do or not do, what course in life to take, whether we are doing the right thing or should be doing something else. All we need to do is pray for the knowledge of God's will for us (and that will always works in our favor) and the power to carry it out. After receiving that knowledge, and feeling that power, we are readily convinced that this is the way to live. It is in no way abrogating responsibility. It is seeing ourselves as connected to universal principles, being on the giving as well as the receiving end of a system of mutual benefit in which nothing is ever lost except trouble and nothing ever gained except joy.

Step Twelve

"Having had a spiritual awakening as the result of these steps, we tried to carry this message to [food addicts], and to practice these principles in all our affairs."

The spiritual awakening is experiencing the strength and serenity that come from changing destructive behavior. When people are suddenly able to do things they couldn't do before, no matter how hard they tried; when they begin to feel life is worth living even though their circumstances may not have changed; when they realize there is more to life than what they thought— much more—they feel an urge to give to others what they have been so readily given themselves. The 12-step program works because people help each other stay in recovery. In fact, recovery is not possible without the Twelfth Step. You may know people who are "dry alcoholics," who remain sober by the white-knuckle method, without AA. They are rarely happy people. Life is just as unhappy as when they were drinking, often worse, because now they have to deal with reality on an hourly basis. The Twelfth Step describes the difference—without a spiritual awakening and the willingness to help others, there is no recovery.

The Twelfth Step does not mean you stand on the corner and proselytize. This is an anonymous program, and it works because it is one of attraction, not promotion. The new person you are will inspire others, not what you tell them. But if there is someone you know who is gaining more and more weight, who looks miserable and acts helpless, don't wait for that person to approach you. Remember the isolation you felt before you sought help. Engage her in conversation. She may open up about her problem, or you might tell her about yours. If she is ready to be helped, you will know. If she rejects help, don't feel you have failed. You have planted a seed.

Practicing the Twelfth Step is a pure form of loving, for it asks nothing in return. Nevertheless, those returns are without measure—in a maturity of outlook, a profound happiness, a circle of deep friends, and a purpose for being alive.

ACTIVITIES FOR DAY TWENTY-FIVE

Assignment One: Writing a Plan for Living

What is your attitude toward change and growth, having come this far? Are you committed to making some changes? Do you feel your reactions to life have changed as a result of having been introduced to the Twelve Steps, and do you know how these changes came about? To help you with these important questions, I encourage you to make some initial preparations. Try listing some of your defects, the attitudes and behaviors that are causing you the most trouble in your life. List some of your assets, too, and incorporate them into your plan for personal growth. What about your new program of spirituality?

Write this material down. Try to be as specific as possible in making your plan for living. *Then live it!*

A DAY IN THE LIFE

Martha I will never forget Chuck as long as I live. I don't even know his last name and don't need to. He is another angel, only instead of wings he has a huge belly. He knocked on my door in my hour of darkest need. I had just spent the worst time I have ever known in a session with my brother. Until today he was the baby and then the cute little boy I took care of and protected from as many blows as I could manage. I took some of those blows myself. That was how I saw myself, dear diary, as his big sister hero, his savior from harm. But how wrong I have been! His words still sting and I can't take them in. I'll write them down and look at them. I AM OBNOXIOUS. HE CAN'T STAND BE-ING AROUND ME, I AM SO OPINIONATED, JUDGMENTAL, CONTROLLING. I NEARLY RU-

*INED HIS MARRIAGE WITH MY INTERFER-
ENCE. IT IS A BURDEN BEING AROUND ME!*
Then the "nobody's" and the "everybody's" started,
and Bob put a stop to it. Keep it to what you alone feel,
he said, and so my brother started in again with a fresh
attack of being madder than I have ever seen him,
bloodshot mad like ma used to get with that wild look
in his eyes. He screams at me, tears streaming down
his face, can hardly get the words out, "But you don't
remember all the times you hit me! Right across the
face! Don't you know that all these years I've been dying to hit you back when you get all self-righteous?"

I can't tell you how deeply I was wounded to hear
this because I know he was telling the truth. I knew at
that moment I HAD hit him—many times—and that
every time I get all upset seeing a little kid get hit on
the street or anywhere, the upset is about what I had
done. Dear diary, I wanted to die.

That was the state I was in when Chuck knocked
on my door. "Can I come in?" he said. "I'm really
hurting."

Sure, I said. I felt honored that he had come knocking on my door with a problem.

When he stepped into the room, I saw that he was
crying. I had seen him cry in group, but these tears were
different. They fell and he kept wiping them away and
every now and then blew his nose, but he never really
told me why he was hurting. Instead, he started telling
me how he identified with me and respected me for
sticking my neck out in places where I wasn't wanted,
and for being true to what I believed. "You're also a
pain in the ass, though," he said, "and I love that part
of you, too." Well, I started bawling like he had complimented me. And then he started bawling. I said, let's
go pour ourselves a nice hot cup of chicken broth and
so we did, only he had a diet soda, and we sat and
talked for a long time. That is, dear diary—I swear to
God—he talked and I listened. I really heard. I didn't

say a single thing about what had just happened to me with my brother and how awful I felt. He talked about himself and how we were alike because he was the oldest child of a violent parent, too, only there were two of them, both alcoholics, and two little kids to protect day and night, and how he never got any sleep, and how he gained weight to be as big as, and then bigger than, his dad. It was a great conversation, and I was secretly proud of myself. I hardly said a thing, and I really heard what he was saying. For a while I even forgot my own problems. I felt light.

But don't think I'm flattering myself over his identifying with me. Chuck and I couldn't be more different. Everyone loves him, and everybody hates me. But that's OK. I happen to like myself somewhat these days, even today. It started to happen when my brother forgave me. He hugged me when he left and said he probably wouldn't be alive today if it weren't for me, and that from now on we could really be close. I feel a tremendous relief coming out of nowhere.

•

DAY TWENTY-SIX

Choosing a Therapist

If you have serious problems, it can be dangerous to think you can deal with them by yourself. Dissatisfaction with life, prolonged depression or anxiety, and a sense of helplessness are all indications of a need to go into therapy. I recommend group therapy for the following reasons: One, defenses are broken down more quickly in group than in individual therapy. For instance, if you are blaming someone else for your problems, it's harder to argue with eight people than it is with an individual therapist, and there are a lot of individual therapists who will *never* challenge your point of view.

In one-on-one therapy a patient can easily get lost in mental abstractions. In a group the focus is on social interaction. Patients relate to each other's feelings, and the process of identification comes out of that. This process will not necessarily happen with individual therapists, particularly if they play a passive role and do not interact with their patients.

Another reason I recommend group therapy is the importance to recovery of a sense of belonging. Although you can get that sense of belonging from a 12-step fellowship, you can also hide out in one. You can get support you need from the fellowship, but no one will ever challenge you as a group will. There, confrontation is part of the growth process, with the therapist acting as a protector and moderator so no one gets scapegoated.

I also recommend group therapy because there is less of a chance for distortion to take place. In one-on-one, you may be taking on a therapist's issues and not even know it. For instance, a woman can end up with a male therapist who has a problem with his mother, who then gives a distorted perception of the patient's mother. Or an anorexic might go to a therapist who didn't think she was underweight because of the therapist's own body-image distortions. Considering how many people have such distortions, I think you're a whole lot safer in a group. There, mirrored in the perceptions of six to eight other people, you have a better chance of learning to see yourself the way you really are.

Here are the qualities I believe are important to look for in choosing a therapist:

TRUTHFULNESS. You need someone who will be direct and honest with you, so you don't have to guess what he or she means. Looking for someone who will tell you the truth is first on my list because it's so difficult for us to see ourselves the way we really are. The perceptions the therapist gives you will not necessarily mean it is "the truth," but at least you have a clear picture of how someone else perceives you, and a reality-based jumping-off place to work from. Some therapists are trained to give you nothing back, but to be a "mirror" on which you are to project your own feelings. I believe it's too easy to conceal ineptitude or indifference behind a mask of noninvolvement, and I prefer therapists who speak their minds rather than parrot back what you have just said, constantly asking you, "What do *you* think?" or (worse) saying nothing at all.

DIRECTION. Find a therapist who is willing to give you suggestions. I believe people should ask for what they need and be specific about what they expect to happen. Then, if the therapist isn't willing to give you direction, cross him or her off your list and shop for one who will. (I give direction by encouraging my patients to take risks and change. Knowing how difficult that is, I understand when they don't, but the choice is still theirs to make when they're ready.)

EXCITEMENT. I've had people tell me they have had therapists fall asleep in their sessions! Look into the eyes of your candidate and see if anybody is home. Look for a certain positive energy. If therapists don't exude a joy for living, I seriously wonder about their ability to help their patients develop one in themselves.

NURTURANCE. You can teach professional techniques to therapists, but you can't teach them to care. I am always disturbed when I meet members of my profession who really don't seem to care about people. Some of them have good insight, but I think it's more important for patients to be accepted and understood than given reasons why they behave in a certain way. I certainly wouldn't choose a therapist who didn't make me feel good about myself. In fact, I would avoid one who didn't at all costs! I value caring and being cared about more highly than anything else, and I believe people intuitively know when someone is nurturing. Quite simply, it feels good to be around such a person. We all know inside when we meet a genuinely caring person. We can feel the energy. Trust your intuition if it's important to you to have a therapist of the nurturing kind.

INTEGRITY. If you discover a therapist who doesn't give everyone in a group equal value but gives preferential treatment based on social status, you have made a wrong choice. Everyone has the right to be treated with dignity, and I wouldn't trust a person who didn't practice that.

Group therapy is usually preceded by an intake interview and anywhere from one to five individual sessions before joining the group. At first, you should expect to feel uncomfortable. Looking at yourself honestly produces a lot of anxiety, so you can't use how you feel about the therapy as an indication of whether it's doing you any good. I tell people to commit themselves to ten sessions. If you just can't take it, at least go for five.

Bonding with a group can be a powerful experience. You may not ever be able to see yourself associating with the people in your group, or even liking them much, but the environment of shared vulnerability has the potential for creating a deeper kind of closeness than can happen in a friendship or even a relationship with a significant person. You are not in a group to cultivate friendships or please others, and that well-defined purpose allows you to focus on discovering who you really are and how to free that person imprisoned within you in order to live, **"happy, joyous, and free."**

ACTIVITIES FOR DAY TWENTY-SIX

Assignment One: What I Need

Draw up a list of the six qualities you need most in a therapist. If you have had previous experiences with therapists, evaluate them. Ask yourself, did the therapist make you feel like you could risk being vulnerable? Did you get direction? Did you lie to him or her? Most important, did you make progress? Then, describe in detail a nurturing person in your life whom you trust. Use the good feelings that person evokes in you as your guide when you seek a therapist.

A DAY IN THE LIFE

Chuck   I have to write down my commencement speech because if I don't, I'll just end up bawling and tongue-tied.

> *I came to this place three weeks ago completely shut down. My life had been reduced to sleep, eat, and work. There was no joy in it. I wanted to make a change but didn't know how to do it. When I came in here, I felt this was my last chance. Instead it's been a real beginning. As I prepare to leave, it's hard to convey the difference in me. It's hard to identify with the helpless, hopeless person who walked in those hospital doors. Today I'm full of hope and energy. I have canceled my cable TV and already hooked up with a hometown meeting schedule. I'm looking for a good therapist, because although I've made great progress here, I know there's further to go, more stuff to work out.*
>
> *But the most important goal has already been won. I know who I am and that I am a good person. I know I can be loved just for who I am. I know that*

because I first felt it from you, and that acceptance of who I really am feels better than anything has ever felt in my life. For that great gift I thank you. We may never meet again after today, but I will never forget you.

•

DAY TWENTY-SEVEN

Recovery

There is a destiny that makes us brothers; none goes his way alone. All that we send into the lives of others comes back into our own.

—Edwin Markham

I like to say that we do the surgery in treatment, but real recovery takes place in the recovery rooms of the 12-step program. Before treatment, food addicts can be seen as victims of their disease. After treatment, if they choose to remain in their addiction, they're no longer victims. They've just sold out. They know there's a way out of their addiction, and for whatever reason, they choose not to follow it. You have now relinquished the right to be a victim and are responsible for making a choice between whether you wish to recover or stay addicted.

I agree with you that it's not an easy choice. Recovery is not a sudden landing. It is a process, and no one ever gets recovered, only remains in recovery. For thousands of years, addicts just died of their addiction, but to me, one of the miracles of the twentieth century is the 12-step program, developed by addicts, for addicts, and run by addicts, for the sole purpose of helping them stay in the state of recovery. The reason it has flourished so phenomenally is simple: It works!

One of the common complaints of the nonaddicted

is that when people join a 12-step program, they stop being addicted to a substance to become addicted to the group. There is some truth to this, for we addicts always do things in an extreme way. However, the need for meetings does not and should not remain at the high-intensity level that is necessary in early recovery. At a certain point, there is life beyond the rooms. During the detoxification phase, the body is still craving the substances it has been denied, the mind is not yet clear, and the unaccustomed state of reality is like a too-blinding light after years spent in a dark place. In this super-sensitive phase, a meeting every day is essential—even more if the discomfort is great.

The first ninety days are a constant struggle, after which there is a period of triumph often called the "pink cloud" of early recovery. But the entire first year is a difficult time during which one priority is enough for anyone to handle—staying abstinent and going to meetings. Everything else should be put on the shelf and no major changes should be made, in jobs, relationships, or geographic moves. The first year is no time to fall in love, because the object of our affection is likely to be just that—an object—upon whom we channel all our thwarted obsessive behavior. Years of failed relationships in early sobriety has resulted in a 12-step rule—no relationships during the first year. Of course, everything is a recommendation in the fellowship. If newcomers follow their own rules, they won't be chastised, and then when they come tearful and devastated to a meeting after the relationship has ended badly, they will be comforted without anyone's admonishing them with an I-told-you-so.

People often ask, "How do I know when I'm in recovery?" If you have to ask, you're not. You can have abstinence without recovery. Abstinence is the opportunity for recovery. When all you're thinking and talking about is food, even if you're not abusing it, and when you're using food to hide who you really are, you're still in the addiction. People in recovery radiate it. They have no secrets to hide. Somebody's home and you're being invited in. They're willing to share what they've got. When you reach that state, you'll know it and so will others.

Another problem that's important to deal with in recovery is rigid thinking. One of the things people in early sobriety ask me the most is, "Do you mean I can't have a piece of cake or a cookie or a fudge brownie for the rest of my life?" I believe that's dangerous thinking. First of all, this is a day-at-a-time program. Secondly, it is this kind of extreme thinking that gets addicts in trouble. People should definitely remain abstinent from all mood-altering foods for a year, but after that, they have enough recovery under their belt to stop thinking in "never again" terms.

To avoid the rigid thinking that characterizes addiction, look for patterns. Take the seasons. They ebb and flow in a fixed way, but no one can predict exactly when summer's going to come. A basic to recovery is to set up a new pattern for a life-style you can live with, things you want to change, and to look at it as a natural force in the evolution of life instead of within the narrower scope of following a diet. We, too, ebb and flow like the seasons. Our moods change from day to day, but we are part of a pattern that has a purpose and a direction. It's not that summer won't come, it just comes in its own time and its own way. If we focus on the patterns, a healthy life-style, and a healthy way of eating, instead of focusing on exactitudes and the rigidity of perfection, we can make life a lot more pleasant for ourselves.

Between three and five years into recovery, people begin to take on larger issues. Many go into therapy to deal with them. They can also expand their identity. The phrase "you are what you eat" is so limiting! You may carry the results of what you eat, but you are much more than that. Be sure you leave this treatment phase with a burning desire to find out who you really are. In the beginning it's important to identify ourselves as food addicts, but we need to go beyond seeing ourselves as people with an addiction to who else we are—sensitive, caring people with imagination, dreams, hopes, and thoughts, with something valuable to offer society because we have no illusions about ourselves.

It's not enough to follow the program. You have to learn to think and act responsibly. Otherwise people are just transferring their dependency from one authority to another authority and never learning to think for themselves and deal with unstructured time. There are people who use the program to avoid what's going on at home. To me that's not recovery.

Recovery is about style. It's about developing a style of living until it works. It's about not being afraid to tell people who you are because *you* know who you are and don't care if others like you because *you* like you. Recovery is about having a love affair with yourself so you can have one with life. It's about being happy, joyous, and free.

I wish you great joy and success in your recovery as I have in mine. If I can do it, you can do it, but none of us can do it alone.

ACTIVITIES FOR DAY TWENTY-SEVEN

Assignment One: Aftercare Worksheet

In the new direction you're traveling, your windshield needs to be much bigger than your rearview mirror. What has happened to you is worth a watchful glance now and then, just to make sure it's not tailgating you in the present, but what lies ahead—today—is your major concern.

What are your chances for staying in recovery? Better than with some diseases, worse than with others: The general statistics are that after treatment for depression with addiction, one third continue to struggle, going in and out of recovery, one third go straight into recovery and stay there, and one third relapse. The statistics for my program are better than the national average. By the number of letters I get from former patients, reporting in glowing terms of their permanent changes, I *know* what we're doing works. I also know a well-worked-out program of aftercare can make all the difference.

You will be playing a new game in recovery, with new players. Baseball is the metaphor of the 12-step program for me. You're congratulated when you hit a home run, encouraged by your teammates. It's a gentle game, it moves at a slow pace with polite and elaborate protocol, and it doesn't hurt. Football is the game we played when we were active in our addictions, and it hurt. For a while—for the next ninety days—you're going to stay away from football fields and football players. You'll tell people you've learned to play a new game. You need to make your recovery the number one priority in your life, because, believe me, **whatever you put before it, you will lose.** It's hard for people who are accustomed to putting everyone else's needs first to make themselves the number one priority, but helping yourself first will make you much better at helping others later.

At our aftercare sessions at Janet Greeson's "Your Life Matters," we form a circle and each person says, "I place my hand in yours, so we can do the things together I cannot do alone," until everyone in the circle is holding hands. You can't recover alone. For the next ninety days, you need a meeting every day. You need to call your sponsor every day. You need to take care of yourself and keep doing all the good things you're doing like regular exercise. If you take good care of yourself, the other things in your life will get taken care of, too, without the usual struggle. You will need to let go of relationships with people who don't respect you. You will need to keep the sickness of self-destructive and negative thoughts from creeping back into your mind. You will need to play the game of life with gentle people who abide by the rules that honor recovery.

At 12-step meetings, seek out the winners—the ones with long recovery who show enthusiasm and warmth—and follow them around. Avoid those who project negativity. They are an energy drain you can ill afford right now. This is no time to go around saving others, even if it does feel good to take the focus off yourself and put it onto someone who needs help even more than you.

You also need a specific plan for your aftercare, with dates and times and places. Fill out the forms in the aftercare worksheets in today's workbook with the kind of determination you have learned you are capable of, but don't get too ambitious. Remember, addiction is about extremes, and your tendency will be to throw yourself into this next step, particularly because you feel so good and powerful. But that way leads to relapse. "Easy does it."

Draw a vertical line down the middle of a sheet of paper. On the right side write the word "Plan" and on the left the word "Goal;" on the goal side you will describe what you want to accomplish, on the plan side, how you are going to achieve your goals. Make these plans as specific as possible, with dates, times, and locations, so you don't get bogged down keeping an impossible schedule later.

Your first goal concerns food and other mood-altering substances. If your goal is to remain abstinent, your plan will specify how you will do so: by attending at least four meetings a week, for example, getting a sponsor, planning your meals, or working on the Twelve Steps. Other items to chart are:

—Family and friends
—Recreation and physical conditioning
—Occupation and education
—Spirituality
—Other

Go over this aftercare plan with someone in the fellowship, preferably your sponsor.

Assignment Two: Self-Evaluation

1. List three positive achievements that you feel you have accomplished in these twenty-eight days, physical as well as mental.
2. List three defense mechanisms that you can now recognize in yourself and some recent examples when using them affected you adversely.
3. List three new behavior patterns you are practicing to substitute for these negative behaviors.

Assignment Three: Balance: Interdependence

One of the new qualities you will be developing in recovery is the ability to balance. As addicts, we were driven by the feeling that we would never have enough. We need to guard against overworking "always" and "never." The ability to achieve equity in a relationship is the greatest balancing act of all. Many addicts participate in relationships as a codependent or dependent. The codependent is a martyr, doing for others at his own expense. He often becomes self-abusive because he feels like he is never giving enough. The dependent in a relationship feeds off his partner, concerned only with getting his own needs met. Both derive their identity from their role in the relationship and feel they are nothing without their partner. Both roles are extreme, both are unhealthy. The following chart gets specific about how far is too far and how much is too much when it comes to relationships.

Interdependent	Codependent	Dependent
Detached compassion	Feels responsible for others	Self-centered
Surrounded by people who are mutually supportive	Surrounded by people who are dependent and needy	Manipulates to get needs met
Able to say no without feeling guilty	Feels guilty if doesn't give	Demanding "You owe me!"
Accepts responsibility for own mistakes; also allows others to be responsible for self	Takes on other's responsibilities	Blames others for failure to be responsible
Sets boundaries and maintains them	High tolerance for emotional pain	Numb due to sedation
Receives as well as gives	Gives to manipulate; gives without receiving	Takes, takes, and takes; gives to manipulate
Gives self permission to act human	Alternates between superiority and inferiority	Acts grandiose while feeling worthless
Focuses on self with inclusion of others	Focuses on others to exclusion of self	Focuses on self to exclusion of others

Assignment Four

Make an "I am" affirmation out of the qualities listed under INTERDEPENDENT in the preceding chart.

Assignment Five: Balance: Role Reversal

This is an exercise in developing your "other side" in order to achieve balance, not to change your opinion. The addict tends to have extreme or blanket opinions. Putting them in a wider context will make the person achieve a more balanced approach, and more likely to find him- or herself in the mainstream rather than in the isolation of having an extreme opinion.

Pick a current news item, one that is the subject of a lot of discussion and on which there are definite differences of opinion. Instead of arguing for your own opinion, write a defense for the opposite side. In the process you may find that no situations are all simplistic black and white, but are likely to have many shades of gray as well.

Assignment Six: Empowered by Criticism

I'll never forget a line delivered by Anthony Quinn in an old movie. It had to do with adversity. Quinn's character said, "My father used to say, 'Those who don't break your back will strengthen it.'" That line held such a powerful message for me. I held on to it, and every time I felt I was being criticized or judged, I recalled those words and realized that the situation, although difficult, was making me a better person. Once I reflected on how the experience was empowering me, it didn't feel so antagonistic. Now, I don't go around looking for people who don't like me, but I'm not afraid of criticism. It actually helps me to be more of who I am.

Reflect on adversities you have gone through. How have they strengthened you?

Assignment Seven: Recovery Affirmation

 —Recovery comes through the healing of the spirit.

 —Recovery comes a little at a time. There is rarely a dramatic healing.

 —Recovery is not a place to be reached or a goal to achieve, but an experience you can choose to be in for the rest of your life.

A DAY IN THE LIFE

Jenny I can't believe tomorrow's my last day. And I never did beat the bataka. I know, it's not required. But still, a part of me wanted to pick it up and just beat and beat and beat that old rubber thing against the floor or the wall or a chair, or anything. I'm just so angry, almost possessed by this burning rage. It's about racism, I guess. I just have never seen the point of getting all upset about it. It's like getting mad at the weather, the fact that it gets cold every winter up north. But maybe some day I can get it out, that rage, so it doesn't live inside me and do me damage.

 Peggy is drawing. She draws the most beautiful trees. You can see them sway in the wind. She says she may be heavy in her body, but her spirit is as light as those willow branches swaying in the breeze. We are getting the last bit of sun before I am out of here tomorrow. It is bright but not hot. I love the way it soaks into me. I will remember this moment next week at the same time—1:30 P.M.—when I will be at work and the heating vent will be blowing hot dry air at me under the drafting table. Peggy's arms are pink. When she draws, she doesn't move a muscle except in her arm and a tiny bobbing of her head. Her eyes go zip to the trees and zip back to the paper, zip up, zip back, guiding her pencil. It's amazing to me that she can do it so fast. It's so happy here. I don't want to leave. I will miss Chuck and Gordon and Peggy and Bob and, yes, I will even miss Martha. She has really endeared herself to me. When she screws up her eyebrows listening to you, it's like she's putting a clamp on her mouth so she can't interrupt and talk about herself or give you advice. It just KILLS her but she does it, but I think she's trying so hard to listen she doesn't hear a thing! Martha and Gordon have an assignment today. She is supposed to teach Gordon something about control, and he's supposed to teach her something about spontaneity. I can hear them arguing on the other side of the building. I know what he's going to try to get her to do because he told me: take off her shoes and socks and wade in the duck pond. Now she's squealing like a teenager at a rock concert. What in hell's going on? Can you believe it? She's in the pond and now the ducks are trying to nip her out of there. Can't miss this!

•

DAY TWENTY-EIGHT

We Don't Have It All Together, But Together We Have It All

Addiction is a disease of isolation. People lose some of their essence by doing too much alone. The light of their spirit is dimmed, and it's difficult to get a sense of who they are. It is their spirit that has become very subdued in reaction to the isolation. In isolation people's view of reality sometimes becomes distorted, and they become starved for nurturance, for that energy of others who care for them. As Barbra Streisand sings, "People who need people are the luckiest people in the world."

Many people come into the 12-step programs dispirited because of prolonged isolation. In the rooms of the many kinds of 12-step programs you will meet a lot of people who are starved for love and nurturance, disconnected and struggling to keep in balance, just like yourself. You may not like some of them. That's all right. You will find yourself drawn to others.

When you complete this twenty-eight-day program, I hope you will find a 12-step room where you feel welcome, and that you will keep showing up, because just showing up is 90 percent of recovery. And although you will be going to meetings to do something for yourself—to get better—you may also find yourself showing up for others, and they may start showing up for you. It is then possible to experience the joyful synergy of people connected by a desire to love, nourish, care, and trust.

You may not find the right room right away, but if you keep looking you will find a place for you—a group to be a part of and to stay connected to on that long and never-ending path of recovery, with its frequent surprises and miracles. We know that we may not ever get it all together, but together we have it all.

=====

ACTIVITY FOR DAY TWENTY-EIGHT

Assignment One: Autobiography

Write your autobiography, beginning with your earliest memory. Emphasize emotions, not facts. Include significant people and events that made you what you are today. Write down the messages about yourself you received from these significant people, and the memories of food connected with feelings that go back to your childhood. Be sure to include secrets you kept, and benchmarks, those revelatory moments when you got a new perspective on your life up to that point. Include the history of addiction in your family on both sides where appropriate, the onset of your addictive behavior, and the progression of your addiction.

At this point, you may not feel you have much to write about recovery, but you have just finished a book that has powerfully affected your capacity for change, provided you have done the necessary work. Reflect on changes you have already made, and how the positive feedback from those changes has encouraged you to continue.

This autobiography is meant to be open-ended. In the weeks and months to come, it will have new meaning for you, and you will want to add to the recovery section. Keep it always. It is a legacy of your courage, and it will increase in value to you as the years go by.

Assignment Two: The Journey Begins

Now you are on your own. I don't mean that now you are alone, but that you "own" who you are, and that person has become your most trusted friend, one you can count on to be both truthful and loyal. Every day you need to give this new voice you have rediscovered within you a forum to express itself. You will still get messages from your complaining mental self, who wants to think and scheme and second guess, or from your physical self with all its wants, but let these incessant voices be quieted for three minutes a day to take in the messages from the other voice, the one who wants to live on a more elevated plane where there is joy and meaningful connection, serenity and truth.

Every night for the next ninety days of your recovery, give this voice the opportunity, perhaps right before bedtime, to express itself. Write in a journal and keep the words flowing for three minutes. Begin with the words, "I feel," and when you get stuck go back to those words. After doing this exercise for a few weeks, you will find that the words will flow readily, and you may be amazed to read what's really going on with you!

Learning to value what our real self has to say is

one of the greatest rewards of recovery. Learning to follow it keeps us on the journey. I hope to meet you there one day.

COMMENCEMENT

I was there for the commencement of Martha, Chuck, and Jenny. The mood was joyous and the room was packed, as it always is, with family, friends, staff, and other well-wishers. Twelve patients sat in a row facing the audience, all dressed up and looking like they couldn't smile enough. After a group song, the ceremony began. The primary therapists introduced each patient one by one, describing what they had been like when they came into treatment and how they had changed. Each patient made a little speech, full of tears and jokes and eloquence, about what they had discovered about themselves. Then members of the audience who were moved to speak expressed their feelings. Believe me, it is always a highly emotional time. Then, as the ceremony drew to a close, we all joined hands in a circle and sang again—a popular song with words we all know, one whose message of love moves us deeply. I go to as many commencements as possible. They are truly a celebration of life, and I believe they bind us to our roots. They are our story—our history.

"Your Life Matters" is not a place, it's an experience. It is not necessary to go into treatment to have it, although the process of recovery is accelerated there. Like the people who come to my treatment centers, you may also be familiar with the hurt and pain that no amount of food, alcohol, relationships, or other obsessions can numb. I hope you have learned during the past twenty-eight days that there isn't any magical solution, but there is the process of recovery. It is slow but it is steady, and you have more help than you realize.

The activities for the twenty-eight days were developed to help you diffuse the pain and hurt of what's eating you. Although I hope that diffusion has begun, you may also be realizing that there is no culminating place, no goal to reach, only a journey of recovery. I have been on that journey for close to two decades now, traveling in the company of the Spirit of God, which is my nourishment. So celebrate the fact that your journey has begun. It's your turn now.

III

Recovery One Day
at a Time

8

One Year Later

Jenny, Chuck, and Martha are still in recovery. Chuck has become the chair of his local 12-step group and is working hard to surrender his need to be everybody's good guy. It's a hard mask to drop because there's so much positive feedback from wearing it. However, Chuck has the social skills to be able to define new limits with people. He's stopped making so many promises and commitments and has learned to say, "Sorry, I wish I could help you but . . ." At first Chuck felt so shaky making this change that he dropped back into his old worrying self, but his wife Jean told him that he'd slipped back. "Please don't do this to yourself," she pleaded. He is fortunate to have such a wise and devoted companion who is also willing to take the actions needed to change herself. Chuck is back on track. He and Jean have learned how to truly enjoy themselves. Their relationship can now deepen as they enter full retirement. Recovery shines on their faces. They have healed and mended the damage that has been done. Chuck likes to tell people, "This program is not for those who need it. It's for those who want it. If you need it and don't want it, you're not going to get it." Need is an abstract to him; want means action. "Change is possible," he says. "Just look at me."

The climate Jenny lives in has also profoundly changed. She, too, now wakes up each morning grateful to be alive. Her obsession for the man who doesn't call has ended like a bad dream. She has made other changes. She has moved to a new neighborhood, changed jobs, and is making new friends.

This year was also marked by Jenny playing the role of maid of honor at the wedding of Alice, her mother. In therapy, Alice discovered the source of her obsession with unavailable men: the buried feelings around the sudden death of her father at the age of four. This mother–daughter case history dramatically illustrates family patterns, unconscious repetitions of our most hidden motivations passed from one generation to another. Granted, Alice's ex-husband was a swell person and a devoted father (at least until his children reached adolescence), but he wasn't the only man in the world. Attractive, outgoing, and charming, Alice didn't stay single long, having made her belated discovery about other fish in the sea.

The adult children of abuse—those who were physically battered, treated with unkind words, or sexually violated—come into treatment with a trauma to find, a vivid, repressed event around which old feelings fester. Children of neglect and abandonment have a different task, for there is no single event to find, nothing vivid, only gray and featureless depression. Jenny still struggles with her feelings of entitlement, that she is allowed to feel as badly as she did about her losses. Before treatment, she did not allow herself to grieve over anything her parents had done because she still idealized them. They had to be all good or all bad, and she couldn't paint them the latter. She unconsciously emulated her mother's message: "Love the man who isn't there." Now that the emulation is conscious, it can be changed. Every now and then she finds herself getting excited over an unobtainable man. For a week she was very interested in a man who told her he was gay. Jenny laughed off her mistake and said, "Can we be friends?" They are. "That's called getting better," Jenny says.

Martha's year in recovery has been the most rocky. Had it not been for her brother, who assisted her in getting a retail job in Seattle and loaned her money to set up a new apartment, Martha would have been stuck in her same graveyard shift service job. Thanks to her brother (who may be making amends for the unkind words he had to say about his sister in session), she is managing an import shop in the Seattle seaport area and enjoying the hustle and bustle and the atmosphere. Still, she is fighting to get back into the teaching profession and saving her money for a potential lawsuit against her previous employers for unfair dismissal.

Martha is a mainstay of her local 12-step group. She has helped save lives there. It is Martha who goes up to newcomers and latches onto them when they waver. It is Martha who calls a person who hasn't been seen in the rooms for a few days. It is Martha who will sit up all night with someone, or go to the hospital with a gift and cards. She is a good soul. Her former self has dropped away. Believe it or not, she is now a woman of few words. One day she quietly let go of the need to control, and after a period of intense panic, she experienced the comfort and joy of the simple state of being. Martha is an essentially practical woman: her attitude about therapy was, "Does it work?" It has worked for Martha. Once she found what worked for her, she did not waver. People who knew the old Martha are amazed by the transformation. What happened to her? they want to know. But Martha doesn't talk much about herself anymore. She doesn't tell, she only shows.

9

Janet's Story

"... What is Real?" asked the Rabbit one day.

"Real isn't how you are made," said the Skin Horse. "It's a thing that happens to you."

"Does it hurt?" asked the Rabbit.

"Sometimes," said the Skin Horse, for he was always truthful.

"Does it happen all at once?"

"You become real. It takes a long time. But once you are Real you can't become unreal again. It lasts for always..."

—from *The Velveteen Rabbit,*
by Margery Williams

I was born in the Red Hook section of Brooklyn, in a working-class Irish neighborhood, as World War Two was coming to a close. My father was in the Army, and my mother was my universe. I was her first child. My earliest memory dates from age four when my life, which had been tranquil up to that point, took an alarming turn. My mother went to the hospital to give birth to my brother, and instead of the few days of life without her I had been prepared to endure, I was told she was sick and would be gone for ten days.

I was taken to my paternal grandmother's house in Queens, which to a child from Red Hook was like going to a foreign country. With her French–German accent, even my grandmother seemed foreign to me. Although she had a glorious garden with every kind of flower imaginable, and a fine house surrounded by soft green grass, my grandmother was cold and rigid. She was of the opinion that her son had married beneath him, and I always had the feeling there was something different about me that couldn't be discussed. Also, having lived by herself for many years, she was not at all comfortable around children, even one she might have approved of more than me.

I had to sleep with her. She had a habit of slathering her wrinkles with Noxzema right before going to bed, and I lay every night feeling as if I were being gassed by the fumes. To this day I can't bear the smell of Noxzema.

Then, when the ten days had finally passed, my grandmother told me my mother was home from the hospital but still too sick to care for me, and an eternity slowly passed while she did nothing but listen to the radio. The favorite thing for my mom and me to do was go to the movies. Finally I got my grandmother to take me to one, where I caused a ruckus, hoping she would think I was so horrible she would take me back to my mother.

My plan didn't work. As the days passed, I grew increasingly fearful that I would never see my mother again. Finally, after three interminable weeks, I was so desperate I decided to end my life. I found a rope and tied one end to the top of the cellar door, the other around my neck, and jumped. My grandmother found me and was so upset she hit me. After that she never let me out of her sight. Although I had rope burns on my neck, she never told anyone what had happened and neither did I. It became a secret.

Although I didn't want to be separated from my mother, she was difficult to be attached to, and more so after my brother came along and I had to share her attention. I can still see her, very obese then and usually alone, lying in bed reading romance magazines. I remember feeling that if I took care of myself, it would be a help to her. My mother never knew the luxury of childhood, for she had nine brothers and one sister and pretty much raised the boys. In spite of her being surrounded by people all the time, I saw her as an isolated, lonely woman.

Although I always carried with me a fear that if something happened to my mother I would die, the message I received from her was clear: *You're a big girl now. You can take care of yourself.* We lived in a housing project, and every morning she would tell me, "Go out and play," but when I went downstairs, I couldn't find any children there because it was too early. One of the benchmarks of my life is standing in the courtyard looking up at hundreds of windows and feeling very alone.

But I could take care of myself. I was a big girl. When I went to kindergarten, my mother walked me to school the first day, a long walk through Coffey Park. After a few days she said, "You can go by yourself now. Get somebody to cross you," so I used to stand on the street corner and wait for some other kids to come along with their mothers to get across the street.

We moved to South Brooklyn when I was in first grade, but I finished out the year in the school in Red Hook, taking a city bus to the old neighborhood for two months by myself. In the process I became a very independent child.

While my mother gave me the message that I could take care of myself, my father gave me another: *Be responsible, work hard, achieve great things.* He did all these things and had a good job working for the Transit Authority as a trainmaster. He was a big, strong man, outgoing and attractive to the women. I can see him at night in his chair, disappearing into one of the six or seven books he read every week. Although he was there, he was absent, and I yearned for contact with him. I thought I would win his love by being responsible, working hard, and achieving great things, but there was no real intimacy between us. I went to the movies once with him when I was nineteen. That's the only thing I can remember ever doing with him, just the two of us.

The thrill of my life, and the most intense source of love, was my maternal grandfather. I was crazy about him. He was brilliant, charming, and a roaring alcoholic. People loved him and took care of him. I actually remember wishing he was my father. I would say that if I ever wanted to be like anyone, I wanted to be like him. I don't ever recall my grandfather working, but I have many fond memories of him cooking meals, in which he took great pride. He loved to tell people how much I ate, and it was an easy way to get his approval. I even ate sardine sandwiches, which would repulse most kids, but I ate them for him.

He loved to take me to all those great Irish bars under the Myrtle Avenue el. I would stand on the bar, singing and dancing, a real little Shirley Temple, surrounded by laughing, approving men, getting money from them, and my grandfather getting drunk on the money and me on the attention. I couldn't get enough of that. On the way home he would always say, "Don't tell your mother where we've been," which made our trips to the bars all the more exciting.

There was another secret we shared that weighed much more heavily on my small mind, and that I knew without his saying a word should never be revealed. "Let's take a nap," he would say. I knew he was doing something wrong, but I loved him so much, and the conflict was intense. He was the only one in my world who seemed exciting to me, and because of our secrets I felt I was special. Without him I was nothing. I was only five or six years old, but I learned to live with the conflict.

The new neighborhood was more friendly and less crowded than the projects: two rows of brownstones with the focus on the street, which belonged to the kids. It was a safe place, and it rang with the noise and laughter of children in every kind of weather. On warm days and nights, grown-ups sat on stoops up and down the street and watched out for us. I was raised by an entire block of neighbors, most of them related to each other, forming a real clan right there in the middle of Brooklyn, and it was a great life.

Along with my Irish relatives and neighbors, there were a lot of Italians on the block, and they liked to cook pasta for me because I was such a hearty eater. One of my favorites was baked macaroni and cheese. Food was an expression of love that worked two ways: the pleasure I gave others because of the large amounts of food I was willing to consume for love, and the approval they gave me for eating it. Of course, I was obligated to eat it all and was glad I had an appetite that was up to the task, since that appetite was emotional, not out of true hunger.

In my family, eating and drinking to excess was a way of life. My mother, my grandmother, and my great-grandmother were all obese. When my great-grandmother died, they had to break a window and take her out like a piano because they couldn't get her through the door. While the women ate, the men drank. There was a lot of violence, a lot of chaos, and always a lot of food, which was highly valued by people who had experienced many long years of deprivation during the Depression and then the shortages of World War Two.

In school I was spirited, a leader, and excelled at everything I did. I channeled a lot of my energy into sports, where I learned to become a team player, and it was a great way to get the attention I craved. There was always part of me that was a maverick, and another part of me that wanted to lead people and be around them. I felt happiest when surrounded by people, but even then, racing to get my teammates out of the prison zone without getting tagged, with kids and babies and grown-ups all around, inside I always felt lonely and bad, a sense of shame I never understood. All I knew was, somehow I would never be enough.

I know today where those feelings came from. My mother and I were bonded in a way I didn't know then, by a man—her father and my grandfather—who sexually abused us. That was the origin of the shame, a mirror image, and the loneliness was bonding with a woman who had never completely bonded with anyone else. Today, having shared our secrets, we *are* bonded, by a love that goes much deeper than our mutual pain. Having been less than the perfect mother I wanted to be, I am now able to embrace her unconditionally. We work together, see each other nearly every day, and share a rich, full life.

But then I didn't understand. I only felt the shame and the loneliness and the belief that I was never enough.

When my father left for work, my mother would say, "Let's order a pizza." It was always the two of us, plus food. We ate well and often. A full meal would be followed two hours later by ordering out Chinese food. My mother was generous but she didn't share. If you wanted a slice, she would buy you a pizza, but she wouldn't give you any of hers. If you wanted one of her M&M's, she would buy you your own bag, a big one. Food was too important to share.

Television became an important part of Brooklyn life in my growing-up years. Although my father was usually too busy reading, he watched *Kraft Television Theatre*. It was the only time the entire family watched television together. I still vividly recall the cheese commercials, the dishes floating magically before our eyes. I would buy the cheese for my mother, and she would make the recipes. To this day I have a great affection for cheese. Maybe it connects me to that time and the presence of my father, his attention diverted from his usual solitary activity to focus with his family on those powerful commercials.

It's strange how many of my most vivid childhood memories are about feelings I had in connection with food. I wanted to be a part of something; connected, bonded. When I went to my maternal grandmother's house, I was always encouraged to raid her refrigerator, but she would tell me, "Save the pineapple juice for Uncle Eddie." Out of spite I would sneak into the kitchen and drink some straight from the can, trying to get away with as much as I could without being noticed. To this day I love pineapple juice and never drink it without thinking about how I had to save it for Uncle Eddie, still wondering: How come I had to save it for him? Was pineapple juice too good for me?

I grew tall, and because of my hyperactivity, I didn't really have a weight problem for many years. I was obsessed with sports, ballet, tap dancing, and never performed any of them in moderation. During summer vacations I played from ten o'clock in the morning until nine o'clock at night. I played basketball with the Police Athletic League and the YMCA and won all kinds of championships.

I excelled in school as well as in sports, although I never, ever studied. I started drinking around the age of twelve, and by my midteens was a real party girl. I loved the euphoria alcohol put me in. A new drink came out called the screwdriver. The first time I tried it, I had about twenty of them and blacked out. From that moment on, I was a vodka baby.

I skipped a grade in high school and graduated when I was fifteen. Instead of going on to college, I wanted to join the Navy. Living close to the Brooklyn Navy Yard, sailors had always been a big part of my life, ever since my bar-hopping days with my grandfather, and I wanted to get a sailor. I didn't want to be an officer because I didn't think they had the fun that real sailors did, and I thought an education would lock me out of that. After graduation, working in the Greenwich Savings Bank until I was old enough to join the Navy, I lived the high life. Although I went out with hundreds of sailors in my teenage years, I had never had sex with them. My mother had explained the facts of life to me at an early age and told me not to trust men. "They'll tell you they love you, but the only thing they're after is your cherry." I really believed it, not just because of my mother's warning, but because I saw that my sexually active girlfriends were always jumping from one man to the other without getting the respect I craved.

As soon as I turned eighteen, I went to the Navy recruiting office, where I was told I had to lose twenty pounds before they would take me. That was my first diet. It was simple: I didn't eat for ten days, danced a lot, and lost twelve pounds. When I went in for my physical, the recruiters were so impressed they figured I would lose the rest in boot camp and inducted me.

As soon as I was approved, I started eating until I reached 190 and I had to get down to 170 to get into boot camp. In boot camp I was put in the Pudgy Platoon with all the people who had to take off weight. When the Pudgy Platoon was marched to chow, we went in the back of the line and got no bread, potatoes, or desserts, just meat and vegetables. I spent a great deal of my time in boot camp negotiating: "If you'll give me your bread and your dessert, I'll do your ironing." There was no way I was going to give up my food.

My job in the Navy was similar to what I had done at the bank because I was really bright when it came to math and accounting. I was in payroll. There was a lot of power in being in disbursing, close to the money. I traveled, to Norfolk, Newport, St. Albans, San Diego. At last I had left behind the reclusive life my mother lived, which I despised. It had always been inconceivable to me that she had never even been to see the Statute of Liberty.

At first everything was great. My life was so exciting—men, alcohol, parties, crazy times, feeling worldly. Everywhere I went I was popular and dated a lot, and because I wasn't the type to just jump in bed with anybody, I had a lot of sustained relationships. Nearly everyone drank a lot, and I certainly didn't believe I had a problem with alcohol, although the trouble I did get into almost always involved alcohol. When I'd be late or fall asleep and get restricted, losing my liberty pass, I'd climb into someone's trunk and get them to drive me out of the gate.

After two intense years of the high life, I began to think my life was deteriorating. My drinking was out of control and I had gained a hundred pounds. I started finding myself in uncomfortable situations with people I didn't want to be with, seedy people. I felt superior to them, that I was lowering my standards, and feared if I stayed in the Navy I would start sinking into a bottomless pit. One night, falling deeper and deeper into this state, I thought of my father and decided my problem was a lack of responsibility. If I was married and had children, I would have to act differently.

Driven by my father's message, I called up a man I had known all my life. He was in the Navy, of course, and seven years older than me. Every time he had come home on leave when I was growing up, we went out together. He soon proposed. I accepted. I knew he loved me, and it didn't matter if I loved him. After all, who else was going to marry me at 268 pounds?

I was twenty years old when I got married. My wedding gown was a size 48, and so heavy it bent the hanger. People told me I had a pretty face, and hearing that always made me feel awful, for it negated the rest of me. Shortly after the wedding, I got pregnant, and my husband was deployed overseas. Suddenly I was alone for the first time, minus my customary social life, soon to be a mother, and without the faintest idea of how to really live. I felt as if I were dying. I had exchanged identities, giving up the party girl for the wife.

Worst of all, I was back in the old neighborhood. My husband's family lived across the street. Between my husband and me, we probably had fifty family members living on the same block, but I was not close to them the way I had been with the people I had been stationed with in the Navy. Like Alice in Wonderland grown too big for her house, I could not fit into that old life anymore. I had seen too much of the world. In spite of the close contact, there was no real intimacy, and I felt trapped.

I went through pregnancy and childbirth without my husband. He was gone for a year and a half. Old feelings of abandonment were tapped into and magnified a hundred times. My misery was so great, my addictions to food and alcohol began to take over my life. The responsibilities of marriage and motherhood had not rescued me, only made my need to alter my state of mind all the more urgent. The alcohol made me feel good, but when it made me feel bad, I used the food to feel good again. When I got sick from drinking too much, I ate to feel better, so no matter how I felt I was either eating or drinking to excess, and my weight mushroomed to 340 pounds. The bigger I got the more invisible I felt, for I had lost my identity under all that fat. I didn't feel I deserved to live and was slowly trying to kill myself.

When my husband finally returned, he got stationed at a Navy base in Lakehurst, New Jersey, and I went with him, thrilled to be out of my old Brooklyn neighborhood. Two years after the birth of Gene, I had another child, Jimmy. On the base I met a childhood friend with whom I used to run around in my party days.

She was also stationed there with her husband. We got together and it was party time all over again.

I have a friend who says a social drinker is someone who every time someone says they want a drink, says, "So shall I." I was like that. I really believed that social drinking was drinking with people, telling myself I didn't have a problem because I never drank alone or in the morning. Also, I never drank at home unless I was having a party, telling myself only alcoholics drank at home.

Although I didn't want to stop drinking, I had a great desire to lose weight. I thought if I were thin, I could get my life back. I went to a doctor on Eastern Parkway in Brooklyn, who treated obesity with shots of pregnant women's urine and a diet of 300–500 calories a day, and lost a hundred pounds in four months. My seven-year marriage had been shaky for some time, and it ended with my weight loss. Shortly thereafter I met Charlie. Unlike my first husband, who was an alcoholic who didn't drink, Charlie was a Marine, an active alcoholic and lots of fun. I loved him and he was crazy about me. He was probably more like my grandfather than anyone I had ever known, not just in looks but in personality, too. I was in heaven, which for me was a place that was exciting, chaotic, and unpredictable.

My daughter, Rosemary, was born in 1970 and we moved to Florida. There Charlie and I had a classic alcoholic marriage. We brutalized each other. He was physically abusive when he was drunk, and I never knew what would upset him. He started combining alcohol with drugs and became even more unpredictable.

Meanwhile, I lost the same hundred pounds three times. I was always either on a starvation diet or putting the pounds back on that I had just lost, faster than I had lost them, plus a few extra. I went on the Stillman diet, I went to Elaine Powers. I went to TOPS, where I frequently took home the pig, given to the person who had lost the least amount of weight that week. I went to Weight Watchers. The instructor told us we had to take the skin off the chicken we ate, and I made a face. She pointed a finger at me and said, "That's why you're fat." I was mortified and told myself, "I'll show that bitch." I lost weight for a little while, but for the wrong reasons.

I exercised like a fiend. I went to all kinds of diet doctors, and most of them gave me pills. Sometimes I'd go to three doctors at the same time and take all the pills, believing that whatever was going to work, if I took more of it, it would work better. One doctor I saw was morbidly obese. He handed me a prescription for pills and said, "These will work for you." I thought, How come they don't work for you then? but didn't say anything, afraid I wouldn't get the pills. I had to have that magic.

But there was no magic. Everything I tried failed. I had become a chronic dieter, either miserable on one or miserable because I wasn't on one. As soon as a diet set up the deprivation pattern, I was kicked into the internal void I had lived with all my life, that hole inside me that made me angry and full of despair. I am convinced that my reaction to that deprivation caused me to be heavier than I would ever have been had I not dieted at all.

When I was at my heaviest, my husband and I took a vacation to the Bahamas and boarded one of those small planes that take you from one island to another. I sat in the back as I did wherever I went, not wanting to be noticed. The plane taxied around the runway several times and then went back to the terminal. As my husband and I started wondering aloud whether there might be some mechanical difficulty with the plane, the stewardess approached us and asked me to move to the front of the plane and lean toward the middle. I was so heavy the plane was off balance, and they couldn't get it off the ground!

I was mortified, and so was my husband. A normal

person would probably have taken a vow at that moment never to binge again. Not me. The first thing I did when I got off the plane was eat. I had to numb out, and I continued to eat my way through the Bahamas, because I kept worrying about how I was going to get back. The humiliation triggered the memory of other similar experiences, like the time I got stuck on a log flume ride in Coney Island because the machinery jammed. By the time I finally made the splash, it seemed as if a cast of thousands had gathered, hooting and clapping. I was dying inside then, too, and went straight to Nathan's and had popcorn, hot dogs, shrimp—anything I coud get my hands on to numb those awful feelings.

After the Bahamas debacle, I went crazy with my eating. I would buy a loaf of Italian bread, make a hero, and eat the whole thing. Sometimes I would just chew my food and not swallow it. Then I discovered if I ate enough jelly doughnuts, I could bring them right back up again. I went to a clinic where I drank a solution, and they pinched and pushed the fat out of you. I was nearly kneaded to death and didn't lose a pound. I tried whatever magical cure I heard of for taking off weight, making pilgrimages from place to place. I was going to have an intestinal bypass but decided not to, because a friend of mine made an appointment first and told me the doctor had warned her there was a 10 percent chance she would die from the operation. I thought, with my luck, I didn't dare risk the odds.

I read in the paper about a woman in Italy who glued her teeth together to lose weight. She lost a hundred pounds, plus her teeth. Then one day I was watching Phil Donahue interview a woman who had lost weight by having her mouth wired shut and drinking regular Pepsi. I was amazed at that, wondering why anyone would waste calories drinking regular soda. Still, I thought the idea was fascinating and decided it was my last resort.

I called a lot of dentists in Orlando. Most of them laughed at the idea and refused. Finally I found an oral surgeon who said he would do it for me. "Do you want to have your jaws wired tomorrow?" he asked. I told him I had to go on a vacation first. I went to New Orleans and Houston and put on another twenty-five pounds.

The procedure was excruciating. Sometimes I wonder whether the doctor didn't make it more painful than necessary as a deterrent. He put wires through my gums on the top and the bottom, attached them to a bar, then wired the two bars together. After three days I was banging my head against the wall, wanting something to hurt more than my mouth did. I took my son to Sea World, thinking that if I was around people, I wouldn't cry. I cried anyway. Then the pain started to subside somewhat, and I started suffering for other reasons. After three weeks of a liquid diet I was crazed. I started pulling at the wires, creating a little hole through which I could stuff food. It would take me hours to eat what I would normally consume in ten minutes.

When I went to the dentist to have my teeth cleaned, I watched him take the wires off in the mirror so I could figure out how to do it myself. It was difficult, because I had to reverse the process I saw in the mirror, but I managed to take them off, binge, and then wire them up again so nobody would know, then pray I wouldn't throw up from all the food I had been eating and choke to death. I knew what I was doing was insane, but I just had to have that food. I couldn't stand what was going on. My drinking increased as my food intake decreased, and I began to deteriorate physically. I ended up with alcoholic neuritis and could hardly walk.

Looking back, I see that period as my bottom. I wanted to die and couldn't, but I didn't want to live. My life was utterly out of control. In desperation I went to yet another overeaters' group, this time at the Orlando civic center. A friend of mine had told me about it, and I went with her and my mother. We went to the wrong location, and by the time we arrived, the meeting had already begun. I sat in the back, taking up two chairs, in the vain hope I wouldn't be seen. It was January and cold, but I was sweating and a nervous wreck. The speaker said to me, "You're late." I cringed and looked around for the diet. There wasn't one. That made me uncomfortable and intrigued at the same time.

The speaker told her story and then started talking about God. An atheist in the meeting started arguing with her, joined by an agnostic and a Jesus freak. I sat in the back on my two chairs, thinking, "What the hell's going on? Where's the diet?" I didn't even know what an agnostic was, and what did God have to do with losing weight? Then another woman, obviously from New York by her accent, spoke about how she had lost 112 pounds—not over and over like I did, but more or less permanently. I decided I didn't like her. She was too aggressive.

As soon as the meeting was over, I said to my mother and my friend, "Let's go eat." We went to a restaurant, stuffed ourselves, and laughed disparagingly at everybody at the meeting, the argument over religion, and the lack of a diet. I couldn't believe what I had witnessed, but I kept thinking about the woman from New York who said she had lost 112 pounds and not put them back on. That kept running through my mind, together with something someone had said about love. It hit home, as I had always connected food and love. And so I went back.

The next week the woman from New York started following me around. "Can I help you? Is there something I can do to help you?" she kept saying. I ignored her. She was the last person I wanted to be around, and I thought she was too pushy. That meeting the topic was feelings, and a lot of people were crying. I started to cry, too, and said to myself, What's happening to me? This is powerful, and when a list came around with people's names and phone numbers, I signed it.

The woman from New York called me every day. She asked me what I was going to eat that day and I wouldn't tell her, so she asked me what I had eaten. I started sharing that with her. She kept pursuing me in spite of my defiance and wouldn't give up on me. Beneath my front was a fearful woman who needed to have someone going after her. The addict in me didn't want to change, but the submerged healthy person in me desperately did, and during that struggle, the woman called me every day.

The addict in me wanted magic, drama, chaos, and extremes, and not a slow process. Going to meetings and talking on the telephone every day was none of what my addict wanted, but there was someone else living inside me who desperately wanted to get better, and I kept going back.

The woman from New York saved my life. Except for that uncomfortable moment at my first meeting when I was accused of coming in late, no one in the group had judged me. I didn't have to look like Twiggy to be accepted by them. I didn't have to look like anybody. I was okay just the way I was.

In that atmosphere of acceptance, I started following instructions, willing to acknowledge the fact that my way obviously wasn't working. It wasn't education about food I needed. I knew what to eat and what not to eat. I needed a change in attitude, and I got that following the program, doing the assignments I was given, and going to meetings. I wanted to live instead of exist, and I knew I wouldn't be doing either for long if I didn't lose weight. There was something in the eyes of the people who went to the meetings that kept me coming back. They were real. I felt closer to some of them than others, but they were all real. They had all been through Death Valley and come out laughing.

I lost a hundred pounds that first year, and fifty

pounds the next. I had experienced dramatic weight losses before, but this time it was different: I kept the weight off, month after month and year after year. Another thing was different: I was learning to like who I was, even when there was three hundred pounds of me, so when I came in contact with my slimmer self, I wasn't terrified of who that person was, as I had been before. It was still just me and I was okay. At a certain point, my intense craving inexplicably went away. I simply didn't need food to make me feel good anymore. I had learned how to do that by valuing and taking care of myself.

Instead of being addicted to food, I became addicted to meetings, and that was okay. After all, I'm an addict, and in the early years of my recovery I was compelled to do something in the extreme. I got extremely active. I became another pushy lady from New York who followed terrified newcomers around, asking, "Is there anything I can do to help you?"

My husband was not happy about my new self. In fact, he was threatened by it. The more weight I lost, the more insecure he became. When I was eating addictively, even though I was miserable, our relationship was comfortable in its familiarity. Because my eating was out of control, I was full of fear and felt powerless, completely dependent on my husband. He earned a good income as a career officer, and I hadn't worked for years. I hated having to count on someone else for financial survival and knew I had to prepare myself for being on my own. I desperately wanted to be responsible for my own life, and I knew education was my only ticket out. Charlie didn't want me to go to college but agreed to my attending motel–hotel school. When I told one of my instructors I was proud of the grades I got, he told me, "You don't belong here. This is nothing to you. You need to go to college."

One year into recovery from my food addiction, my perceptions of what I was capable of accomplishing changed, and I gave up alcohol. That was too much for my husband to handle. He had often told me he would leave me if I got sober, and he made good on his threat. We had been living and raising three children on an income of $22,000 a year. That dropped to $5,000 a year once he left. I got very sober. I had a little money stashed away, plus a savings account for my children's education. That plus a job waitressing paid the bills.

As painful as that time was, my children and I were closer than ever. When my addictions were controlling me, I had been irritable a lot of the time and it was easy to take out my anger on them. Sometimes if they dropped a crumb on the floor, I would turn into a maniac. Gene told me he was grateful for my changes. When I was active in my addictions, he wouldn't bring any friends to the house because he never knew when I might go off on a tangent, and he was afraid to be around me most of the time. After I went into the fellowship, he told me he'd rather be around me than anyone in the world. A lot of the anger had been an expression of my feelings of powerlessness, but flying into a rage had no place in my new perception of myself. Getting close to my children was one of the greatest gifts of my new life. My strength infused them, which in turn increased my own, and we all benefited from the changes I had made.

The emptiness I had lived with all my life was beginning to fill up with something so precious I can only venture to put a name on it. Spirituality is one, God is another, or maybe it was my soul, but those are all abstract concepts that can be argued *ad infinitum* with no increase in understanding. What is unarguable is the quality of the people who came into my life during this time.

There is a story about a skeptic who got lost in the wastes of Alaska. About to die from exposure, he prayed to a God he didn't believe in for help. Soon afterward an Eskimo came by and brought him back to civilization. Later the skeptic chided God, "Why didn't you help me when I was so desperately in need?" and God replied, "What do you want from me? I sent you an Eskimo, didn't I?" Rather than get involved in spiritual abstractions, I prefer to focus on tangibles— the Eskimos who turned up at this crucial point in my life to sustain, encourage, and love me when I was still unable to have kindly feelings toward myself.

One of my Eskimos is Terry Lamonde. I love the image of the crusty old mama she likes to portray. Her qualities of intensity and vivid individuality were what first struck me about her, but deeper than her style was a commitment to really *be* there for others. When I was with her I experienced what it was like to receive unconditional love, and it was so powerful I knew I was in contact with someone important, who had something to teach me about how to live life. I had no idea Terry was an Eskimo when I met her, but I have learned to identify them since as the people who come into your life when you are ready to learn something. She taught me to focus on what was really important and to take risks in spite of my fears. She believed in me so strongly that I developed an equally strong desire to believe in myself.

Margaret was another Eskimo. She kept urging me to go to college. "You help so many people," she said, "I really think you should become a psychologist." She even offered to baby-sit so I could go, and that impressed me. Marie, my sponsor, was another. She was not a bright woman, "just another alcoholic" to some, but to me she was special. She taught me how to give love and just be. She had an aura of simplicity about her that I really needed to understand. I felt like her daughter. There were many others, and their message was all the same: You can do it. I didn't believe in myself, but I believed in them.

I enrolled in the University of Central Florida

shortly after I stopped drinking. I hadn't been in a classroom since the age of fifteen, half my life ago. I was still so obese I couldn't fit behind the desks, and my thoughts were so scattered I was afraid I had damaged my brain with alcohol. Full of fear, I was apologetic for just being there. I felt terribly isolated as I kept quiet and tried not to bother anybody. As awful as I felt, I went, day after day, until those feelings of inevitable failure began to dissipate, and a few successes began to validate my right to be there.

Then I really took off. Always an extremist, I became supercharged. Working part-time as a waitress and carrying as many as twenty-four hours a semester, I managed to earn a four-year degree in psychology in less than three years. Not even a bout with cancer of the cervix was able to slow me down. Instead of congratulating me on my degree, Marie urged me to go on and get a master's. By this time, I had come to believe that I could do anything, and I went on to get an advanced degree. I wanted it for myself, but I also wanted it for Marie, who was dying of cancer. Toward the end, when she was too ill to go out, I brought about ten people to her house and we had a meeting. The topic was acceptance. She sat in a chair and talked about her fear of dying alone, and there was so much love in her I knew she couldn't really die. The feelings we all had for her wouldn't stop when her body ceased to function.

I brought her to the hospital the following Monday. Four days later I woke up, knowing Marie was waiting for me to come to her so she could die, and I avoided going to see her. Suddenly, walking aimlessly around a shopping mall, I said to myself, What are you doing here? and ran to my car. When I walked into her hospital room, she was in a coma, but I knew she knew I was there. I told her, "I'm here with you," and held her and talked to her until she died in my arms. Marie's legacy to me was to go out and be an Eskimo, to give to others what she had given to me: her simplicity and her unconditional love. She lives through me.

While getting my master's degree, I worked part-time in the Navy's alcohol rehab program, a joint venture with the University of West Florida. With my usual zeal, I became first a facilitator, then a screener, next a coordinator, and finally a trainer of facilitators. Because I was addicted to food as well as alcohol, I wanted the center to treat both, and tried to convince the director to begin to look at food as an addictive substance. He was reluctant at first, having worked hard just to get alcoholism recognized as a disease, and was concerned that bringing in food addiction would dilute the program. I understood his reluctance. No treatment centers were treating food addictions at the time, and the Navy is not known to be an institution that encourages maverick thinking. Compliance is what they value. But I had been a maverick all my life and I persisted. I felt like a pioneer. I was a pioneer.

I believe you can educate someone who abuses a substance into recovery, but not an addict. I had been educated plenty—by my humiliation in the airplane that couldn't take off, by the horrors of finding ways to eat after having my mouth wired, and by a thousand other painful lessons—and so I knew no amount of education got me to stop behaving addictively. I argued that treatment had to go beyond detoxifying the body and educating the mind. Addiction is also a disease of the emotions, and no amount of intellectual understanding will treat them in any meaningful way. My logic was, that instead of focusing on the substance, the external disease, we should focus on the whole person—the body, mind, emotions, and spirit—helping people break through their defensive, self-destructive behavior patterns to get them to change what they were doing in their life *today*, to give them tools that would allow them to create an identity for themselves and set them free.

My persistence paid off. I opened up an alcohol rehab center that was therapeutic and 12-step oriented. Unlike other treatment centers I had heard about where people were shamed and humiliated, I stressed love, acceptance, safety—all the things I had discovered I needed in order to change. It worked. People did change. Like me, they dared to take risks and turn their lives around. The program was so successful it became a model for other treatment centers.

When I first came into the fellowship, I was taught that fear and faith can't live in the same house. I bought that idea, and I used to worry when I was afraid that I was doing something wrong. Now I believe I will probably always have fear in my life. When I speak from a podium in front of thousands of people, I'm absolutely petrified. Sometimes I'm afraid just to get up in front of a group of patients. I'm not as articulate as I would like to be, and sometimes I beat myself up about that.

I've learned to think of fear as part of my nature and have made the choice either to act with fear, or to fear and take no action. Over the years, I've always chosen the action. I tell myself fear is just another feeling and act in spite of the way I feel, and that is what has made me successful. When people protest by saying it doesn't feel good to be afraid, I say, it doesn't matter. Acknowledge the fear and do what you know is right in your heart. Good things will come from that.

When I opened the first center in 1986, my heart was pounding. Most people are advised not to launch a new business unless they've got the security of a substantial amount of capital to float on. My capital was more the size of a rowboat than a cruise ship, and that made me full of fear. I was told by the bank that I might get the money I needed to start operating the center in a few months, but I couldn't wait that long and borrowed $100,000 on my own. A friend of mine had received $50,000 that had been willed to her, and her grateful husband added another $50,000 to that. Then I went out and got every kind of credit card I could get my hands on, over twenty of them, and that's how I financed the center. Most people wouldn't do that because they need to feel secure. I took my insecurity and did it anyway.

Buddy also played an important part in motivating me to start the center. We were born on the same day, and when he came into the program at five hundred pounds, I became his close friend. I was also close to his wife and daughter. Buddy was an artist and did beautiful graphics and artwork for a conference we worked on together. Just before the conference, he died. He was one of the numerous people in the program we had lost from their addiction that year, and I was angry that we had all these treatment centers for alcoholism but there wasn't any really structured help for food addiction. I took that anger and used it as energy to motivate myself to make a difference, to deal with something that had always been neglected by society, and to help other people like my beloved Buddy live long, full, and useful lives.

In opening up the centers my motivation has never been to make money. I used the same approach to financial success that I do with food addiction: In order to conquer the latter you do not try to conquer it, and in order to be a financial success, you do not try to make money. I have made a lot of money, and I spend it just as fast. Money is not a priority. God, family, and friends are my priorities. Good begets good that comes back to me as more good—it's contagious!

There's a saying that I have adopted as one of my guides through life: "Die young—as late as possible." Youthfulness to me means the ability to take active participation in creating one's own destiny, to be willing to risk failure and rejection, and to be resilient when the failure and rejection inevitably occur. The incredible life force within us is available to anyone who wishes to tap into it. But it often becomes blocked by depression, which inhibits our ability to be absorbed in what's happening in the present and causes us to dwell on the past.

Boredom is an early indication of a slip back into depression, and at 42 percent, the most frequent cause of relapse—more than social situations or emotional issues! Boredom is about not really living life. It's about falling into a passive form of existence, a desire to be entertained rather than to actively entertain life's great and often unexpected possibilities. Sometimes people in early recovery slip into the habit of watching too much television, which only increases their boredom. Next thing you know, they start succumbing to all those tantalizing food commercials and decide to eat to relieve their boredom. Unless they pull themselves out of their lethargy into purposeful activity, they can fall right back into the addictive cycle.

People who make a contribution and have a purpose in life are never bored. There's so much to do! When I was on the sidelines of life, controlled by my addiction, I didn't know what my purpose was, or have a clue as to the kind of contributions I could make. Today, there are not enough hours in the day to do everything I want to do.

Yet, I swear to you, there's nothing unique or special about me. If I can do it, you can do it. God gives all of us gifts. Some put gifts in a closet, but I relish the gifts I get, use them to maximize my contribution to life, and have received so much real nourishment in return.

I am a model of recovery. Today I really believe I'm God's kid and that has made all the difference.

The loneliness I have carried around with me all my life is still with me at times, but most of the time I really feel as if my cup runneth over. I possess an energy I know is more than the sum of my parts, which I don't try to analyze. I know people who are married or in a relationship who experience a more severe kind of emptiness than I do. When that void begins to ache, I see the little girl within me who didn't understand and I embrace her. There is only one person in the world who can help her, and that's God and me. When I am nurturing her, I am not angry or filled with fear. I feel good about being able to take care of myself, I don't have to give my all to a man, and I feel good about that, too. For some reason men find that intriguing. Maybe they realize there's a part of me they're never going to get. They sense the power of my boundaries and that attracts them.

My mother and I have a unique relationship in that she's my best friend, and I enjoy being with her. I'm aware how rare that is between mothers and daughters and am grateful for it. We live in proximity but maintain our private lives. We work together and help each other solve our daily problems and know that no matter what happens we will be there for each other. We've grown beyond mother–daughter to mainstays.

My deepest and strongest relationships are with my three children. They each give me something special. Gene, my oldest, gives me his 100 percent acceptance. He loves and understands me, and I him. When he was in high school, he always scored low on intelligence and aptitude tests, and his high school counselors laughed at him when he said he wanted to go to college. I told him, "Gene, you can do anything. You're going to college." I drilled into him that his test scores didn't matter, and I told him my story about how intelligence is like a glass of water: People can have half a glass, a quarter of a glass, or a full glass. It doesn't matter how intelligent they are, it's what they do with what they have.

Gene went to college, first to Loyola, then Notre Dame, and he graduated from Tulane. He's very successful today with a career in the Navy.

Jimmy is a lover and an old soul. He looks mischievous with his long hair and dancing eyes, a second-generation hippie. His face reveals his wisdom, that he knows what's really important. He's a musician who plays electric guitar, and he's going to be famous one day. I know that he will always be there for me, no matter what, and I for him.

Rosemary lights up my life. She radiates joyfulness. If I spend just a few minutes in her presence, she energizes me, and I see that happen with others just as much as with me. She inspires people and also accepts them, just as they are. Her message is simple but clear—she wants them to be happy. All three of my kids are a strong part of the ebb and flow of my life. I give to them, but they also give back to me, and I think that's important. I get the impression from a lot of parents that we should just give and give to our kids and not expect anything back, but that's stressful, and I see this one-sidedness particularly in addictive families. I believe the flow of love has to go both ways so that everyone is constantly replenished.

I have learned to live in the middle spectrum of emotions, where addicts are so uncomfortable, because I find that there I can remain on a more even keel. That way the intensity isn't there when I make mistakes, either. Other people are often devastated when things go wrong, but I'm usually not. For instance, in alcoholism treatment I believe that I don't get them drunk and I don't get them sober. When there are accolades about the treatment and people pay compliments, I don't pick them up. The other side is, when something goes wrong, I don't pick that up, either. I just don't need external validation because I get that from within.

I save my excitement for recovery. I know I'm God's kid and that gives me a zest for living. I know He has better plans for me than I could ever dream up. I know that I'm a messenger, an Eskimo, and that my spirituality doesn't belong to me but works through me. I just keep showing up and doing what I believe I've been put on this earth to do. In my more than fifteen years of recovery, I've come to believe in the saying that it's not the end of the journey that matters, it's the journey that matters in the end. I travel light. I enjoy the trip. I'm still excited about recovery. I'm real, and that's all that matters.

Janet Greeson, Ph.D.

Affirmation for the
Rest of My Life

———

I am not my body
I am free
I am as God created me
I am part of a community
I am safe and strong
In my own company
For I am not my body
I am free.

The Twelve Steps
of
Alcoholics Anonymous

1. We admitted we were powerless over alcohol—that our lives had become unmanageable.
2. Came to believe that a Power greater than ourselves could restore us to sanity.
3. Made a decision to turn our will and our lives over to the care of God *as we understood him.*
4. Made a searching and fearless moral inventory of ourselves.
5. Admitted to God, to ourselves, and to another human being the exact nature of our wrongs.
6. Were entirely ready to have God remove all these defects of character.
7. Humbly asked Him to remove our shortcomings.
8. Made a list of all persons we had harmed, and became willing to make amends to them all.
9. Made direct amends to such people wherever possible, except when to do so would injure them or others.
10. Continued to take personal inventory and when we were wrong promptly admitted it.
11. Sought through prayer and meditation to improve our conscious contact with God *as we understood Him,* praying only for knowledge of His will for us and the power to carry that out.
12. Having had a spiritual awakening as the result of these Steps, we tried to carry this message to alcoholics, and to practice these principles in all our affairs.

Reprinted by permission of Alcoholics Anonymous World Services, Inc.

For information about Janet Greeson's
"Your Life Matters"
Please call 1-800-515-1995

Janet Greeson's

Your Life Matters

Consulting Services for Matters of the Heart

Author of *It's Not What You're Eating,
It's What's Eating You*

FOOD FOR
♡ LOVE ♡

HEALING
THE FOOD,
SEX, LOVE
& INTIMACY
RELATIONSHIP

JANET GREESON, Ph.D.

Unlike diets and other fads, this powerful recovery
program can help you change your approach to
food *permanently*.

BOOKS THAT HELP
TO SOLVE YOUR
PROBLEMS